T0263575

Quality Outcomes and Costs

Editors

DEBORAH DELANEY GARBEE
DENISE M. DANNA

CRITICAL CARE NURSING CLINICS OF NORTH AMERICA

www.ccnursing.theclinics.com

Consulting Editor
JAN FOSTER

June 2019 • Volume 31 • Number 2

ELSEVIER

1600 John F. Kennedy Boulevard • Suite 1800 • Philadelphia, Pennsylvania, 19103-2899

http://www.theclinics.com

CRITICAL CARE NURSING CLINICS OF NORTH AMERICA Volume 31, Number 2
June 2019 ISSN 0899-5885, ISBN-13: 978-0-323-68230-5

Editor: Kerry Holland
Developmental Editor: Laura Fisher

© **2019 Elsevier Inc. All rights reserved.**

This periodical and the individual contributions contained in it are protected under copyright by Elsevier, and the following terms and conditions apply to their use:

Photocopying
Single photocopies of single articles may be made for personal use as allowed by national copyright laws. Permission of the Publisher and payment of a fee is required for all other photocopying, including multiple or systematic copying, copying for advertising or promotional purposes, resale, and all forms of document delivery. Special rates are available for educational institutions that wish to make photocopies for non-profit educational classroom use. For information on how to seek permission visit www.elsevier.com/permissions or call: (+44) 1865 843830 (UK)/(+1) 215 239 3804 (USA).

Derivative Works
Subscribers may reproduce tables of contents or prepare lists of articles including abstracts for internal circulation within their institutions. Permission of the Publisher is required for resale or distribution outside the institution. Permission of the Publisher is required for all other derivative works, including compilations and translations (please consult www.elsevier.com/permissions).

Electronic Storage or Usage
Permission of the Publisher is required to store or use electronically any material contained in this periodical, including any article or part of an article (please consult www.elsevier.com/permissions). Except as outlined above, no part of this publication may be reproduced, stored in a retrieval system or transmitted in any form or by any means, electronic, mechanical, photocopying, recording or otherwise, without prior written permission of the Publisher.

Notice
No responsibility is assumed by the Publisher for any injury and/or damage to persons or property as a matter of products liability, negligence or otherwise, or from any use or operation of any methods, products, instructions or ideas contained in the material herein. Because of rapid advances in the medical sciences, in particular, independent verification of diagnoses and drug dosages should be made.

Although all advertising material is expected to conform to ethical (medical) standards, inclusion in this publication does not constitute a guarantee or endorsement of the quality or value of such product or of the claims made of it by its manufacturer.

Critical Care Nursing Clinics of North America (ISSN 0899-5885) is published quarterly by Elsevier Inc., 360 Park Avenue South, New York, NY 10010-1710. Months of issue are March, June, September, and December. Business and Editorial Offices: 1600 John F. Kennedy Blvd., Suite 1800, Philadelphia, PA 19103-2899. Periodicals postage paid at New York, NY and additional mailing offices. Subscription prices are $160.00 per year for US individuals, $406.00 per year for US institutions, $100.00 per year for US students and residents, $206.00 per year for Canadian individuals, $510.00 per year for Canadian institutions, $230.00 per year for international individuals, $510.00 per year for international institutions and $115.00 per year for Canadian and international students/residents. To receive student/resident rate, orders must be accompanied by name of affiliated institution, data of term, and the *signature* of program/residency coordinator on institution letterhead. Orders will be billed at individual rate until proof of status is received. Foreign air speed delivery is included in all *Clinics* subscription prices. All prices are subject to change without notice. **POSTMASTER:** Send address changes to *Critical Care Nursing Clinics of North America*, Elsevier Health Sciences Division, Subscription Customer Service, 3251 Riverport Lane, Maryland Heights, MO 63043. **Customer Service: 1-800-654-2452 (US and Canada); 314-447-8871 (outside US and Canada). Fax: 314-447-8029. E-mail:** JournalsCustomerService-usa@elsevier.com **(for print support) and** JournalsOnlineSupport-usa@elsevier.com **(for online support).**

Reprints. For copies of 100 or more of articles in this publication, please contact the Commercial Reprints Department, Elsevier Inc., 360 Park Avenue South, New York, New York, 10010-1710; Tel.: 212-633-3874, Fax: 212-633-3820, and E-mail: reprints@elsevier.com.

Critical Care Nursing Clinics of North America is covered in *MEDLINE/PubMed (Index Medicus), International Nursing Index, Nursing Citation Index, Cumulative Index to Nursing and Allied Health Literature, and RNdex Top 100.*

Contributors

CONSULTING EDITOR

JAN FOSTER, PhD, APRN, CNS
Formerly, Associate Professor, College of Nursing, Texas Woman's University, Houston, Texas; Currently, President, Nursing Inquiry and Intervention, Inc, The Woodlands, Texas

EDITORS

DEBORAH DELANEY GARBEE, PhD, APRN, ACNS-BC, FCNS
Associate Dean for Professional Practice, Community Service and Advanced Nursing Practice, Professor of Clinical Nursing, LSU Health New Orleans, School of Nursing, New Orleans, Louisiana

DENISE M. DANNA, DNS, RN, NEA-BC, CNE, FACHE
Chief Nursing Officer, University Medical Center New Orleans, New Orleans, Louisiana

AUTHORS

CYNTHIA BAUTISTA, PhD, APRN, FNCS
Associate Professor, Egan School of Nursing and Health Studies, Fairfield University, Fairfield, Connecticut

AARON CARPENTER, DNP, Mdiv, CPNP
Director, Advanced Practice Nurses, Nemours Al Dupont Hospital for Children, Wilmington, Delaware

BENITA N. CHATMON, PhD, MSN, RN, CNE
Instructor of Clinical Nursing, LSU Health New Orleans, School of Nursing, New Orleans, Louisiana

BENNETT CHERAMIE, BSN, MSN, RN, CHCiO
Vice President of Information Systems, General Health System, Baton Rouge, Louisiana

CLAUDIA DER-MARTIROSIAN, PhD
Associate Director, Veterans Emergency Management Evaluation Center, US Department of Veterans Affairs, North Hills, California

ARAM DOBALIAN, PhD, JD, MPH
Director, Veterans Emergency Management Evaluation Center, US Department of Veterans Affairs, North Hills, California; Professor and Director, Division of Health Systems Management and Policy, The University of Memphis School of Public Health, Memphis, Tennessee

LEANNE H. FOWLER, DNP, MBA, AGACNP-BC, CNE
Assistant Professor of Clinical Nursing, Director of NP Program and Adult-Gerontology Acute Care NP Program Coordinator, Doctor of Nursing Practice Graduate Program, LSU Health New Orleans, School of Nursing, New Orleans, Louisiana

ALICIA R. GABLE, MPH
Senior Project Director, Veterans Emergency Management Evaluation Center, US Department of Veterans Affairs, North Hills, California

ANNE REID GRIFFIN, MPH, BSN, RN
Clinical Investigator and Senior Project Director, Veterans Emergency Management Evaluation Center, US Department of Veterans Affairs, North Hills, California

KELSEY HALBERT, MSN, RN, CNL, SCRN, CNRN
Nurse Navigator, Yale New Haven Hospital, New Haven, Connecticut

JOLIE HARRIS, DNS, RN, CAS
Faculty, LSU Health New Orleans, School of Nursing, New Orleans, Louisiana

CATHERINE HAUT, DNP, CPNP, CCRN, FAANP
Coordinator of Nursing Research and Evidence-Based Practice, Nemours Al Dupont Hospital for Children, Wilmington, Delaware

JESSICA LANDRY, DNP, FNP-C
Assistant Professor of Clinical Nursing, Primary Care Family NP Program Coordinator, Doctor of Nursing Practice Graduate Program, LSU Health New Orleans, School of Nursing, New Orleans, Louisiana

LINDA LEDET, DNS, APRN, PMHCNS-BC
Assistant Professor of Clinical Nursing, LSU Health New Orleans, School of Nursing, New Orleans, Louisiana

CATHY MAHER-GRIFFITHS, DNS, MSHCM, RN, RNC-OB, NEA-BC
Vice President of Quality, Woman's Hospital, Baton Rouge, Louisiana; Instructor of Clinical Nursing, Graduate Program, LSU Health New Orleans, School of Nursing, New Orleans, Louisiana

JANE MERICLE, MHS-CL, BSN, RN, CENP
Chief Nurse Executive, Nemours Al Dupont Hospital for Children, Wilmington, Delaware

SHERRI MILLS, MSN, RN
Chief Nursing Informatics Officer, LCMC Health, New Orleans, Louisiana

MELISSA F. NUNN, MSN, CPNP-PC
Instructor of Clinical Nursing, Pediatric NP Program Clinical Coordinator, Children's Hospital New Orleans, LSU Health New Orleans, School of Nursing, New Orleans, Louisiana

JENNIFER RATCLIFFE, DNP, MSN, RN
Clinical Division Nurse Coordinator, Patient Care and Quality

LINDA ROUSSEL, PhD, RN, CNL, FAAN
Visiting Professor, DNP Program Director, Texas Woman's University, Denton, Texas

BRANDY WILLIAMS, MSN, RN
CCRN-K Clinical Outcomes & Projects Coordinator, Cardiac and Critical Care Services

Contents

Preface: Improvement of Quality Outcomes and Cost of Health Care　　　ix

Deborah Delaney Garbee and Denise M. Danna

Electronic Health Records and Use of Clinical Decision Support　　　125

Sherri Mills

In 2009, the Health Information Technology for Economic and Clinical Health (HITECH) Act was signed into law. Along with this initiative came the push for meaningful use of the electronic health record. Clinicians, information technology professionals, and informaticists must partner to create evidence-based clinical decision support models to guide patient care using tools such as structured computerized physician order entry, order sets, templates, alerts, and reminders. Clinical decision support should be used to improve the quality of patient care and compliance with regulatory standards, while inherently following a provider's workflow.

Telehealth Use to Promote Quality Outcomes and Reduce Costs in Stroke Care　　　133

Kelsey Halbert and Cynthia Bautista

Stroke can cause severe disability and death in the adult population. Many stroke patients do not have access to resources required to provide a timely diagnosis and treatment. Telestroke can provide these patients the accurate diagnosis and appropriate treatment they require. Telestroke has been linked to improved functional outcomes in the treatment of acute ischemic strokes. There are several barriers to providing a telestroke service, such as licensure and liability, reimbursement, technology, and financial issues. It is important to recognize these barriers and begin to implement strategies to overcome them. Telestroke use is cost-effective by reducing stroke complications and disabilities.

Impact of a Mobility Team on Intensive Care Unit Patient Outcomes　　　141

Jennifer Ratcliffe and Brandy Williams

Mobility for critically ill patients has been found to be safe, beneficial, and feasible, although a culture of immobility prevails in many adult intensive care units (ICU) because of staffing challenges and lack of physical therapy and occupational therapy involvement. Clinical practice guidelines recommended early mobility for ICU patients to improve long- and short-term outcomes. Addition of a mobility team to the licensed physical therapy and occupational therapy staff and interprofessional ICU team improved patient outcomes and staff satisfaction, and reduced facility cost related to employee injuries.

Leadership's Impact on Quality, Outcomes, and Costs　　　153

Linda Roussel

In the move to increase effectiveness in valued-based organizational cultures, mindfulness leaders are charged to create environments that foster curiosity and creativity in uncertain times. Mindfulness increases situational awareness and improved communication enhances a culture of safety and better patient outcomes. Mindfulness leadership matters, providing effective ways to communicate and collaborate with others. Results matter, increasing the ability to sustain improvement through increased awareness, and enhancing healthy work environments and joy in the workplace. This article provides useful tools, strategies, and tips for mindful leaders and facilitates greater impact on improved patient and employee outcomes.

Health Care Information Technology: Moving from Support to Performing Care   165

Bennett Cheramie

Technology in health care has spanned several decades. Over the last 60 years, technology has grown to include all parts of health care, with latest advancements around EMR platforms, analytics, and interoperability. EMR platforms are costly, and adoption was slow until the Federal Government developed incentives for adopting technology; this created a boom of health care IT platform adoption. This increased the amount of health care data available. EMR, IT platform, and analytics are used to measure disease processes against best practice, drawing parallels between practice and outcomes. Health care technology is now necessary to provide quality care to patients.

Maternal Quality Outcomes and Cost   177

Cathy Maher-Griffiths

The quality of maternal care in the United States is receiving increased attention due to rising rates of severe maternal morbidity and maternal mortality when compared with other developed countries. Many of these events are considered preventable. The lack of adoption of evidence-based maternal patient safety bundles and tool kits requires immediate attention. Maternal levels of care described by the American Congress of Obstetricians and Gynecologists requires increased focus so that women are in the appropriate facility to receive care. Perinatal care management, integrated behavioral health, and preconception care should be considered a preferred methodology to achieve optimal maternal outcomes.

Pediatric Quality Metrics Related to Quality and Cost   195

Catherine Haut, Aaron Carpenter, and Jane Mericle

The institution of pediatric quality in health care has grown in the past decade but continues to evolve. Children's health care emphasizes the importance of maintenance of health and prevention of illness, which can be measured based on immunization rates, routine or scheduled well care, and early intervention. Pediatric quality measures and indicators have become the basis for payment of services and a true goal to value. Designing processes such as pay-for-performance models, volume-based care, and coordination of care assist in assuring that children receive high-quality health care.

Geriatric Trends Facing Nursing with the Growing Aging   211

Jolie Harris

This article expands on the Gerontological Society of America leaders' work to explore challenges facing healthcare providers in preparing for an aging population. Traditional medicine and models of care may no longer meet complex patient needs. Older patients present with multifaceted issues while living longer with chronic health conditions. The changing environment requires a cross-disciplinary perspective. Changes in reimbursement are in the early stages of implementation and will be used to evaluate measurable outcomes. Preparing to care for this population can only occur with enough health professionals and expanded use of advance practice nurses. Health improvement is economically advantageous.

Treatment and Outcomes in Adult Designated Psychiatric Emergency Service Units   225

Linda Ledet and Benita N. Chatmon

The United States is experiencing a mental health crisis. Access to psychiatric care is drastically declining. Designated psychiatric emergency services (PES) units can provide specialized psychiatric care to patients in crisis. Patients receive immediate, focused psychiatric assessments in a safe environment along with treatment and stabilization with appropriate disposition. Designated PES units foster improved patient clinical outcomes and higher satisfaction rates for psychiatric patients in crisis than traditional emergency departments.

Nurse Practitioners Improving Emergency Department Quality and Patient Outcomes   237

Leanne H. Fowler, Jessica Landry, and Melissa F. Nunn

Emergency departments across the United States struggle to balance the overutilization of emergency services. Nurse practitioners (NPs) practicing in emergency departments improve quality indicators leading to the increased efficiency, timeliness, and effectiveness of care. NPs providing emergency services improve multiple national metrics, such as door-to-provider time, patient satisfaction, diagnostic test ordering, and left without being seen rates. NPs should be aware of the positive impact they make on the quality of care. NPs should monitor and trend patient outcomes they directly effect. More research is needed to identify ways NPs can continue to improve the quality of emergency services provided.

Hospitals Providing Temporary Emergency Department Services in Alternative Care Settings After Hurricane Sandy   249

Anne Reid Griffin, Alicia R. Gable, Claudia Der-Martirosian, and Aram Dobalian

This article reports findings of a qualitative study describing how the US Department of Veterans Affairs cared for vulnerable veterans after Hurricane Sandy while medical center was closed for an extended period. This experience highlights how vulnerable patients continued to need care. Hospital preparedness planning efforts focus primarily on sheltering in place and evacuation. Research is needed to identify how hospitals provided temporary emergency services in alternative settings to inform practical guidance. Hospital planners should anticipate that their most vulnerable patients will continue to need emergency care. Viable solutions should be considered to meet immediate and long-term patient needs.

CRITICAL CARE NURSING CLINICS OF NORTH AMERICA

FORTHCOMING ISSUES

September 2019
Cardiothoracic Surgical Critical Care
Bryan Boling, *Editor*

December 2019
Psychological Issues in the ICU
Deborah W. Chapa, *Editor*

RECENT ISSUES

March 2019
Interventions for Cardiovascular Disease
Leanne H. Fowler and Jessica Landry, *Editors*

December 2018
Neonatal Nursing
Beth C. Diehl, *Editor*

SERIES OF RELATED INTEREST

Nursing Clinics of North America
http://www.nursing.theclinics.com

THE CLINICS ARE AVAILABLE ONLINE!
Access your subscription at:
www.theclinics.com

Preface

Improvement of Quality Outcomes and Cost of Health Care

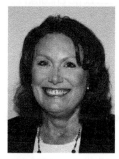
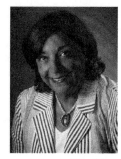

Deborah Delaney Garbee, PhD,   Denise M. Danna, DNS, RN, NEA-BC,
APRN, ACNS-BC, FCNS   CNE, FACHE
                          Editors

Nurses are using data hand in hand with evidence-based practice, bundles, clinical practice guidelines, and various delivery care models to provide patient-centered care and yield improved outcomes. The addition of data analytics holds promise for identification and early intervention to improve outcomes. Data and health care informatics are part of the health care fabric today and essential to guide and document improved patient outcomes and decreased costs. All specialties and settings are held accountable for patient outcomes, and with Medicare Access and CHIP (Children's Health Insurance Program) Reauthorization Act (MACRA) and Merit-based Incentive Payment System (MIPS) requirements, financial impact in the form of penalties when quality metrics are not met compounds increased cost of poor outcomes.

This special issue of *Critical Care Nursing Clinics of North America* includes 11 articles with perspectives on diverse topics related to quality outcomes and cost of health care, including initiatives aimed at improved patient outcomes and decreased costs. Mills sets the stage with an article on the use of electronic health records, computerized physician order entry, and clinical decision support systems, which are embedded in health care workflow. Halbert and Bautista discuss telestroke practice with associated improved functional outcomes, barriers, and reimbursement issues. Ratcliffe and Williams present the outcomes of an intensive care unit Liberation Initiative and formation of a mobility team on patient outcomes, staff satisfaction, and reduced cost. Leadership's impact on quality, outcomes, and cost is presented by Roussel. Mindfulness leadership is discussed along with its impact on a culture for improvement, safety, and effectiveness. Cheramie focuses on the evolution of health care

Crit Care Nurs Clin N Am 31 (2019) ix–x
https://doi.org/10.1016/j.cnc.2019.04.001
0899-5885/19/© 2019 Published by Elsevier Inc.

information technology, big data, data analytics, the shift from volume to value, the impact of MACRA and MIPS, and what it all means to population health outcomes.

Maher-Griffiths presents maternal patient safety bundles and tool kits and subsequent impact on maternal quality outcomes, incidence of maternal mortality, and cost. Several causes of maternal morbidity and mortality are discussed (hypertensive disorders of pregnancy, infections and sepsis, and postpartum hemorrhage) as well as the Maternal Early Warning System. Haut, Carpenter, and Mericle review pediatric quality metrics and present outcomes from value-based care at a large children's hospital system in four states. They report improvement in 23 of 24 pediatric quality metrics. Harris discusses Interdisciplinary Syndrome Care in response to increases in the geriatric population with multiple chronic conditions and what is described as multiple geriatric syndromes, including a "tsunami "of frailty. Ledet and Chatmon describe treatment options and outcomes of adult patient care in designated psychiatric emergency service units. Fowler, Landry, and Nunn provide insight into emergency department nurse practitioner quality outcomes, for example, increased patient satisfaction, reduced wait times, reduced length of stay, and cost-effectiveness. Griffin, Gable, Der-Martirosian, and Dobalian describe their experience of providing temporary emergency department services to veterans after Hurricane Sandy. The authors offer suggestions for disaster planning that includes immediate and long-term patient needs.

Quality and costs of health care have long been a critical issue, with much debate among regulators, politicians, and the health care industry for years. Some authors suggest that the association that exists between health care quality and costs is not fully understood or supported in the literature. This special issue of *Critical Care Nursing Clinics of North America* provides an interesting perspective on the issues.

Deborah Delaney Garbee, PhD, APRN, ACNS-BC, FCNS
Community Service and
Advanced Nursing Practice
Louisiana State University Health–
New Orleans, School of Nursing
1900 Gravier Street, 4A21
New Orleans, LA 70112, USA

Denise M. Danna, DNS, RN, NEA-BC, CNE, FACHE
University Medical Center New Orleans
2000 Canal Street
New Orleans, LA 70112, USA

E-mail addresses:
dgarbe@lsuhsc.edu (D.D. Garbee)
denise.danna@lcmchealth.org (D.M. Danna)

Electronic Health Records and Use of Clinical Decision Support

Sherri Mills, MSN, RN

KEYWORDS

- Electronic health record • Electronic medical record
- Computerized physician order entry • Clinical decision support

KEY POINTS

- Electronic health records provide advantages such as increased availability of patient information, improved interdisciplinary communication, enhanced continuity of care, legibility, improved documentation, reduced duplication, and improved speed.
- Computerized physician order entry within the electronic medical record improves patient safety by reducing medication errors and providing clinical guidance when entering electronic orders by use of prompts and alerts.
- Evidence-based clinical decision support when coupled with the use of an electronic health record can guide the clinical practice of providers and clinicians toward meaningful use and compliance with quality metrics.

INTRODUCTION

According to The Office of the National Coordinator for Health Information Technology (ONC), Health Information Technology "makes it possible for health care providers to better manage patient care through secure use and sharing of health information."[1] They describe the advantages of electronic health records, including efficiency, safety, reliability, and cost savings as well as using meaningful use standards to achieve the highest benefits of the use of an electronic health record.[2] The efficacy of an electronic health record goes beyond the sharing of patient information, although having complete patient information does improve clinical decision making. Increased availability of patient information, improved interdisciplinary communication, enhanced continuity of care, legibility, improved documentation, reduced duplication, and improved speed are other advantages.[3] The use of tools such as computerized physician order entry (CPOE) and clinical decision support (CDS) can go a step further to drive clinical decisions when they are based on clinical evidence and implemented

Disclosure Statement: The author has nothing to disclose.
LCMC Health, 3401 General De Gaulle Drive, New Orleans, LA 70114, USA
E-mail address: sherri.mills@lcmchealth.org

correctly. This review takes a look at these tools and the benefits, risks, and considerations for the clinician.

BACKGROUND

In 2009, the Health Information Technology for Economic and Clinical Health (HITECH) Act was signed into law. This act was designed to "promote the adoption and meaningful use of health information technology."[4] Along with the HITECH Act came financial incentives for providers and institutions who adopted the use of qualifying electronic health record systems.[5] The early adopters of this technology were faced with challenges of poorly designed software with common complaints of point and click medicine, but the drive for patient safety and data aggregation pushed this program forward.[5] The Centers for Medicare and Medicaid Services (CMS) along with the HITECH Act supported meaningful use of this new technology through priorities such as improving safety, quality, and efficiency; engaging patients in their care; improving coordination of care, population health, and information security.[6] The technology boom saw many hospitals and physician offices implement the use of electronic health records, but this was only the very first part of what was intended to be meaningful use. The ability to share records across platforms still challenges health care providers today as does the functionality within the electronic health record. Although designed to improve safety and quality, implementing an electronic health record takes stamina and diligence to identify system weaknesses and opportunities to improve.

COMPUTERIZED PHYSICIAN (PROVIDER) ORDER ENTRY

Computerized physician order entry (CPOE) is defined by the CMS as "the provider's use of computer assistance to directly enter medication orders from a computer or mobile device. The order is also documented or captured in a digital, structured, and computable format for use in improving safety and organization."[7] Computerized physician order entry has been touted as a means to improve patient safety by reducing errors and as a way to save money by guiding order entry.[8] The prescription of the medication is most frequently done electronically using CPOE. Prescription and administration of medication is an important facet of health information technology both inside the hospital and in the clinic and other settings. A study published in 2006 conducted by Brigham and Women's Hospital reported that the implementation of CPOE resulted in tens of millions of dollars of savings over the course of 10 years by providing guidance for prescribing medications as well as preventing adverse drug events.[8] A 2014 review by Nuckols and colleagues[9] concluded that CPOE reduced adverse drug events by more than 50%, demonstrating a strong relevance to improving patient safety. Review of the literature yields many examples of how computerized order entry can and does improve the prescription of medications, whether it be for condition-based dosing, weight-based considerations, or to prevent redundancies and errors. Computerized order entry is not perfect; despite best design and clinical guidance, prescription errors can be made. Singh and colleagues[10] reviewed errors where providers deviated from the structured decision support guardrails, resulting in inconsistencies or even conflicting information within a medication order. This study found that among the identified errors with free text inconsistencies, about 20% "could have resulted in moderate to severe harm" to the patient.[10] The findings highlight that there is an opportunity to improve the design and build of computerized order entry to avoid this type of error.[10] Other errors from CPOE can result from needed software improvement rather than system work arounds.

In a pediatric setting, the entry of patient weight is vital for calculating drug doses, and in one study produced significant findings where the entry of medication orders were allowed without the presence of body weight.[11] More than 30% of the sample required pharmacy intervention for the absence of a recorded body weight followed by frequency and dosage information for drug orders.[11] The findings of such reviews support the additional need for review of technology design as well as collaboration among the user community to identify these trends, work with information technology to identify system fixes, and better training and support for the users of the technology systems.

Computerized physician order entry is one way to guide the practitioner in making decisions as well as navigating the complex electronic order entry process. Combining CDS and CPOE into useful sets of orders can take order entry a step further in attaining quality and safety goals. With well thought out and designed CDS, order sets can provide a layer of sophistication that is unattainable with standard single-order entry. One study also demonstrated a reduced cognitive burden on physicians when using order sets.[12]

CLINICAL DECISION SUPPORT

Clinical decision support tools were identified by the Institute of Medicine (IOM) as a vital function of an electronic health record in 2003.[13] The ONC defines CDS as a set of tools "to enhance decision making in the clinical workflow" and can include alerts, guidelines, order sets, templates, and summaries.[14] Further, CDS can be looked on as "a sophisticated health IT component. It requires computable biomedical knowledge, person-specific data, and a reasoning or inferencing mechanism that combines knowledge and data to generate and present helpful information to clinicians as care is being delivered."[14]

The most widely used and studied types of CDS come in the form of medication safety alerts incorporated into electronic prescribing or ordering systems. Data readily support the efficacy of CDS systems in the areas of medication ordering and reminders because these do not require complex algorithms to support, and typically the data are readily available to support these decisions, but this is basic functionality and certainly does not reflect the potential of CDS systems on clinical outcomes.[15] Outcomes research on medications alerts indicated that they reduced the likelihood and severity of adverse drug reactions.[16] Medication alerts, however, have been found to have high levels of overrides. Research on negative physician attitudes toward alerts for medication safety have identified them as intrusive to workflow and a major contributor to "alert fatigue".[17] A retrospective study by Topaz and colleagues[18] found a 4.4% increase in drug allergy overrides, stressing the need for more accurate allergy alerts to help reduce override rates and improve alert fatigue.

Clinical decision support is meant to take large aggregates of information, compile them, and present them to the clinician to make best practice decisions about patient care.[19] It is imperative that CDS is designed with high specificity to ensure high user acceptance and utilization.[20] Alert format must also be considered. Not surprisingly, the literature showed that an automatic on-screen display of prompts rather than on-demand prompting is best to guide patient outcomes; requiring the user to respond to the prompt showed little difference in the patient outcome.[19]

Clinical decision support in the information technology framework uses software to compare patient data against a database with developed parameters to generate recommendations. These recommendations should be based on best practice or evidence-based practice. The *American Journal of Nursing* defines evidence-based practice as "a systematic approach to problem solving for health care providers, including RNs, characterized by the use of the best evidence currently available for clinical decision making, in order to provide the most consistent and best possible care to patients."[20] Using this evidence and systematic approach, clinical practice guidelines are developed.

Clinical practice guidelines are "systematically developed statements to assist practitioner decisions about appropriate health care for specific clinical circumstances."[20] These guidelines form recommendations for clinicians in the management of patient care, and as designated by the IOM, should be supported by a systematic review of evidence.[21] Although clinical practice guidelines are supported by evidence to improve patient outcomes, there are inherent challenges to adoption.[20] According to a 2001 IOM report, it takes an average of 17 years for new knowledge and evidence to be applied to practice, and even then it is sporadically adopted.[21] This IOM report also challenged improvements to reduce silos and to create care systems focused on care that is safe, effective, patient-centered, timely, efficient, and equitable. Providing effective care is based on evidence and is provided consistently across the spectrum.[21] Even in 2001, when this report was written, it underscored the potential that information technology assisted in this process by providing that consistency. Beyond CDS, the American Medical Informatics Association described adaptive CDS as constantly evolving from re-evaluation of current clinical research, but stated that this evidence should be accessible, current and "machine interpretable" to stay up to date with current literature.[19] Evidence-based practice should be compared with local practice-based evidence; as identified in the article, if locally variable parameters affect the clinical decision algorithm, then those parameters should be incorporated into the local CDS model as well.[19]

Much of the CDS for nursing has centered on care plans and nursing diagnosis, or on evaluation actions that were (or were not) documented rather than a guide to nursing clinical decisions.[22] An electronic health record can expose hidden deficiencies in documentation and through CDS, can guide or even force the use of correct processes and adherence to policies.[3] Nurses recognize the value in clinical reminders for things such as guiding care planning, but there should be a balance so that the triggers do not become a hindrance.[23] The use of alerts "should consider both the evidence for potential clinical outcomes and the features that will fit best into workflow and be accepted by the end users."[18]

With good design, a CDS program can be successful. A 2005 evaluation of a CDS system for use with clinical practice guidelines in the treatment of pressure ulcers revealed the benefits of better knowledge of managing patients with pressure ulcers, better consistency in treatment, and improved communication with the interdisciplinary team.[24] Patient benefits and improvements in care are realized when systems monitor and detect changes in a patient's condition and improve communication with the interdisciplinary team.[25] There are, however, challenges with implementing a CDS system, which include the time to implement new guidelines and to learn the technology, as well as difficulties with the computer system itself.[26]

Current trends have expanded to meet the needs of the nurse in clinical decision making and treatment of patients. A CDS system can provide functionality around alerts (allergies), reminders (restraint order renewal), clinical practice recommendations, nursing diagnosis support, surveillance (tracking Zika), disease prevention (annual PAP smear test), disease management, and medication management (titration dosage).[25] Another good use case for CDS systems is in the area of fall risk assessment and prevention. Duke University Hospital implemented a CDS model within EPIC to alert staff when a fall risk assessment was not performed according to policy and when an appropriate plan of care was not initiated based on a fall risk category. During the study, charting compliance for assessment and implementation of the fall plan of care was improved. Although the documentation improved during this particular study, the clinical outcomes showed no improvement as demonstrated by no change in patient fall rates.[26]

Although the desired effect of a CDS system is to improve patient outcomes, as demonstrated by the Duke University study, this is not always the case. In addition, the presence of a CDS system does not always mean that the clinical staff will use it as designed. Reportedly, nurses tend to rely on CDS when they are new to their role, but with experience, their use of the system is mainly as a system of "double checking," and they rely on their own experience as a primary means of decision making.[27] Some nurses report that these alerts and guidelines control and stifle professional nursing judgment, and although sometimes they can guide quality, when poorly designed they can actually conflict with their experienced opinion.[28] Additional challenges around electronic reminders or alerts include timeliness and accessibility of patient information in support of CDS systems, but these should be reviewed for improvement from a technology and software design perspective.[29]

When evaluating any CDS system, the 5 rights of the system should be used: (1) right Information – clinical knowledge, clinical practice guidelines, and evidence-based algorithms; (2) right people – practitioners, interdisciplinary team, and patient require information to make decisions; (3) right format – alerts, prompts, order sets, templates, information buttons to present decision data; (4) right channels – incorporating the electronic health record, portals, and mobile technology; and (5) right time – pinpointing the time to present the information in the decision-making process that makes the most sense.[30] When these 5 rights are met and the clinician receives patient-specific, relevant information that does not impede care or require additional time and effort, practitioners are satisfied with the CDS system. When the technology exerts more time and energy and restricts actions such as expensive tests and medications, it can be seen as interference with clinical judgment.[31]

When the technology is burdensome or high frequency, clinicians can also suffer from alert fatigue. A study by Sidebottom and colleagues,[23] found that clinicians reported reasons for not using CDS system tools included distrust of data, lack of relevance, too much information, lack of training, information outside of workflow, lack of actionable items, and intrusiveness of pop ups. Interesting feedback from the study was that nurses wanted to be given the opportunity to "do the right thing" before getting a notification that it was not done, reinforcing the importance of timeliness of information to the clinician. The need to incorporate alerts into clinician workflow must be underscored and demonstrates the need to involve end users in the design, training, and implementation phases.[23] Because all nurses do not have the education and technical skills to evaluate the usability of an electronic health record, informatics nurse specialists can play a vital role in assessing clinical applications. The informaticist can assist technical staff in the design of clinical information systems joining nursing science, computer science, and information science and use informatics principles to evaluate system feasibility and improve usability.[32,33]

Clinical decision support systems are important to clinicians but can be leveraged by the patient to explore relevant and evidence-based clinical information to assist in collaboration with their health care provider.[19] The American Medical Informatics Association recognized the importance of a patient, provider, and information technology partnership where a virtual structure for health care and information delivery provides more interactive tools to personalize care.[31] With the continued prevalence of patient portals coupled with biosensors and fitness applications, the demand for health and medical information and advice and decision support will grow.[29]

SUMMARY

The evolution of health care information technology, driven by the HITECH Act of 2009, is only beginning. Through use of intuitive CDS systems, mobile technology, and medical devices that can communicate inherently with the patient record, there is vast potential to improve the quality and speed of patient care. These improved outcomes and the data that support them can, in turn, drive improvements in population health and disease prevention as well.

REFERENCES

1. The Office of the National Coordinator for Health Information Technology (ONC). website. Available at: https://www.healthit.gov. Accessed January 26, 2019.
2. What are the advantages of electronic health records? The Office of the National Coordinator for Health Information Technology (ONC). Available at: https://www.healthit.gov/faq/what-are-advantages-electronic-health-records. Accessed January 26, 2019.
3. Robles J. The effect of the electronic medical record on nurses' work. Creat Nurs 2009;15(1):31–5.
4. HITECH act enforcement interim final rule. Available at: https://www.hss.gov/hippa/for-professionals/special-topics/hitech-act-enforcement-interim-final-rule/index/html. Accessed December 20, 2018.
5. Gold M, McLaughlin C. Assessing HITECH implementation and lessons: 5 years later. Milbank Q 2016;94(3):654–87.
6. Centers for Disease Control and Prevention. Meaningful use 2018. Available at: https://www.cdc.gov/ehrmeaningfuluse/introduction.html. Accessed December 21, 2018.
7. CPOE for medication orders. Available at: http://www.cms.gov/Regulations-and-Guidance/Legislation/EHRIncentivePrograms/down-loads/1_CPOE_for_Medication_Orders.pdf. Accessed December 27, 2018.
8. Kaushal R, Jha AK, Franz C, et al. Return on investment for a computerized physician order entry system. J Am Med Inform Assoc 2006;13(3):261–6.
9. Nuckols TK, Smith-Spangler C, Morton SC, et al. The effectiveness of computerized order entry at reducing preventable adverse drug events and medication errors in hospital settings: a systematic review and meta-analysis. Syst Rev 2014;3: 56.
10. Singh H, Mani S, Espadas D, et al. Prescription errors and outcomes related to inconsistent information transmitted through computerized order entry: a prospective study. Arch Intern Med 2009;169(10):982–9.
11. Alhanout K, Bun SS, Retornaz K, et al. Prescription errors related to the use of computerized provider order-entry system for pediatric patients. Int J Med Inform 2017;103:15–9.
12. Committee on Data Standards for Patient Safety, Board on Health Care Services, Institute of Medicine. Key capabilities of an electronic health record system: letter report. Washington, DC: The National AcademiesPress; 2003. Available at: http://www.nap.edu/catalog.php?record_id=10781. Accessed December 30, 2018.
13. Khanna R, Yen T. Computerized physician order entry: promise, perils, and experience. Neurohospitalist 2014;4(1):26–33.

14. Clinical decision support. The Office of the National Coordinator for Health Information Technology (ONC). Available at: https://www.healthit.gov/topic/safety/clinical-decision-support. Accessed January 2, 2019.
15. Garg AX, Adhikari NK, McDonald H, et al. Effects of computerized clinical decision support systems on practitioner performance and patient outcomes: a systematic review. JAMA 2005;293(10):1223–38.
16. Weingart SN, Simchowitz B, Padolsky H, et al. An empirical model to estimate the potential impact of medication safety alerts on patient safety, health care utilization, and cost in ambulatory care. Arch Intern Med 2009;169(16):1465–73.
17. Ahearn MD, Kerr SJ. General practitioners' perceptions of the pharmaceutical decision-support tools in their prescribing software. Med J Aust 2003;179(1):34–7.
18. Topaz M, Seger DL, Slight SP, et al. Rising drug allergy alert overrides in electronic health records:an observational retrospective study of a decade of experience. JAMA 2016;23(3):601–8.
19. Van de Velde S, Heselmans A, Delvaux N, et al. A systematic review of trials evaluating success factors of interventions with computerised clinical decision support. J Am Med Inform Assoc 2017;24(2):413–22.
20. Pravikoff DS, Tanner AB, Pierce ST. Readiness of U.S. nurses for evidence based practice. Am J Nurs 2005;105(9):40–51.
21. Institute of Medicine. Crossing the quality chasm: a new health system for the 21st century. Washington, DC: National Academy of Science; 2001.
22. Anderson JA, Willson P. Clinical decision support systems in nursing: synthesis if the science for evidence-based practice. Comput Inform Nurs 2008;26(3):151–8.
23. Sidebottom A, Collins B, Winden TJ, et al. Reactions of nurses to the use of electronic health record alert features in an inpatient setting. Comput Inform Nurs 2012;30(4):218–26.
24. Clark HF, Bradley C, Whytock S, et al. Pressure ulcers: implementation of evidence-based nursing practice. J Adv Nurs 2005;49(6):578–90.
25. Piscotty R, Kalisch B. Nurses' use of clinical decision support: a literature review. Comput Inform Nurs 2014;32(12):562–8.
26. Lytle K, Short NM, Richesson R, et al. Clinical decision support for nurses: a fall risk and prevention example. Comput Inform Nurs 2015;33(12):530–7.
27. Dowding D, Randell R, Mitchell N, et al. Experience and nurses use of computerised decision support systems. Stud Health Technol Inform 2009;146:506–10.
28. Ernesäter A, Holmström I, Engström M. Telenurses' experiences of working with computerized decision support: supporting, inhibiting and quality improving. J Adv Nurs 2009;65(5):1074–83.
29. Marshall AP, West SH, Aitken LM. Preferred information sources for clinical decision making: critical care nurses' perceptions of information accessibility and usefulness. Worldviews Evid Based Nurs 2011;8(4):224–35.
30. Borum C. Barriers for hospital-based nurse practitioners utilizing clinical decision support systems: a systematic review. Comput Inform Nurs 2018;36(4):177–82.
31. Greenes RA. Clinical decision support. The road to broad adoption. 2nd edition. London: Academic Press; 2014.
32. Rojas C, Seckman CA. The informatics nurse specialist role in electronic health record usability evaluation. Comput Inform Nurs 2014;32(5):214–20.
33. Kaplan B, Brennan PF. Consumer informatics supporting patients as co-producers of quality. J Am Med Inform Assoc 2001;8(4):309–16.

Telehealth Use to Promote Quality Outcomes and Reduce Costs in Stroke Care

Kelsey Halbert, MSN, RN, CNL, SCRN, CNRN[a],*,
Cynthia Bautista, PhD, APRN, FNCS[b]

KEYWORDS

- Telehealth • Telestroke • Telemedicine • Stroke • Outcomes • Cost

KEY POINTS

- Use of telestroke can increase access to acute stroke care in neurologically underserved areas to improve stroke care.
- Improving functional outcome in acute stroke patients is one important quality outcome that can occur with the use of telestroke.
- Telestroke practice can be cost-effective, improve continuity of care, shorten hospital stays, and avoid unnecessary stroke patient transfers.

INTRODUCTION

Stroke can cause severe disability and death in the adult population. When an ischemic stroke occurs, there is a need to administer intravenous thrombolytics within a defined treatment window in order to significantly improve patient clinical outcomes. Many stroke patients do not have access to the resources required to provide a timely diagnosis and treatment. Telestroke can provide these ischemic stroke patients the accurate diagnosis and appropriate treatment they require, thus promoting quality outcomes and reducing costs.

STROKE AND USE OF TELESTROKE

Stroke is the fifth most common cause of death and ranks first as the leading cause of disability in the United States.[1] For many years, the gold standard in the treatment of acute ischemic stroke has been thrombolytic therapy with intravenous alteplase. Functional outcomes have been shown to improve when thrombolytic therapy is

Disclosure: The authors have nothing to disclose.
[a] Yale New Haven Hospital, New Haven, CT 06510, USA; [b] Egan School of Nursing and Health Studies–Fairfield University, Fairfield, CT 06824, USA
* Corresponding author.
E-mail address: rkelsey.halbert@ynhh.org

administered within 3 hours of symptom onset.[2] Despite this, it is estimated that only 3.7% of eligible patients receive this therapy.[2] One contributing factor is that many of these stroke patients live in rural areas where acute stroke care is not readily available. Approximately 61 million Americans are considered underserved regarding access to specialty medical care.[3] In the United States there are roughly 4.0 neurologists per 100,000 people who provide care for more than 700,000 acute strokes annually.[4] As a growing number of neurologists opt out of call coverage for acute stroke and other neurologic emergencies, the gap between supply and demand widens and a greater number of patients become underserved. State and local regulations that require hospitals to provide emergency call coverage to be recognized as an acute stroke–capable or primary stroke center also contribute to the provider gap. As a result, many patients who present to community hospitals with stroke symptoms have to be transferred to a comprehensive stroke center. Transferring patients is expensive, labor-intense, and time consuming; delays created by such a transfer might preclude thrombolytic and/or endovascular therapies because the patient might arrive outside of the treatment window or irreversible brain damage might have already occurred.[5] The estimated total cost of stroke in the United States in 2009 exceeded $36 billion resulting from health care expenses and lost productivity.[6] Stroke does not affect the nation evenly; rural areas experience a 20% higher stroke-related death rate than urban areas.[6] Telestroke provides an effective solution for providing rural, community, or underresourced hospitals with on-demand access to acute stroke expertise.

Two models of telestroke exist: an off-site stroke specialist uses digital technology to communicate with on-site health care providers who are treating patients at a spoke facility that lacks stroke expertise, assisting with diagnosis and treatment including administration of intravenous alteplase; and a spoke hospital provider receives guidance from a stroke specialist at a hub hospital regarding diagnosis and treatment, but the patient can be transferred to the hub facility if a higher level of care is warranted.[5] In the first model, the teleneurologist is located anywhere in the country, whereas in the second model, the teleneurologist is at a primary or comprehensive stroke center nearest the spoke hospital.

QUALITY OUTCOMES OF TELESTROKE

The teleneurologist can visualize, assess, and converse with the patient as if they were in-person at the bedside, while at the same time review clinical and diagnostic results, developing an individualized treatment plan that takes into account the patient's health history, stroke risk factors, current presentation, and anticipated outcome.[7]

Telemedicine has been recommended by the American Stroke Association and the American Academy of Neurology as a strategy to increase access to acute stroke care and rapid acute stroke evaluation.[8] Spoke hospitals participating in a telestroke network have access to vascular fellowship trained neurologists for an immediate audiovisual consultation; this relationship with an academic hub site fosters ongoing education and formal processes for clinical improvement.[8] Quality outcomes of telestroke utilization (eg, **Box 1**) can occur when this real-time consultation provides timely assessment, accurate diagnosis, and possibly effective treatment.

Rapid recognition and an accurate diagnosis are critical elements of acute stroke care. Because many conditions can mimic the symptoms of acute stroke, the ability to rapidly and accurately differentiate between stroke and stroke mimic is challenging for physicians without neurologic expertise. Delays in diagnosis and failure to diagnose acute stroke limit the use of proven therapies, such as intravenous alteplase. Telestroke provides neurology specialists at a comprehensive stroke center (hub) with

> **Box 1**
> **Quality outcomes of telestroke utilization**
>
> Timely assessment
>
> Accurate diagnosis
>
> Effective treatment
>
> Improved functional outcomes
>
> Reduced morbidity and mortality

the data necessary to assist the bedside physician at a community hospital (spoke) with stroke-related decision-making for patients who initially present to rural or under-resourced facilities. Remote image transmission of a neurologic assessment is as valid as a face-to-face examination by a stroke neurologist and has been shown to shorten the time to complete a stroke patient's evaluation when compared with traditional methods of stroke diagnosis.[3]

Ischemic strokes account for approximately 87% of all acute strokes. Selected patients are good candidates for intravenous alteplase, a thrombolytic agent that can help restore blood flow and potentially reverse or prevent disability if administered within the guideline-recommended time window. The more quickly this agent is administered, the greater the chances for recovery with minimal or no neurologic deficits.[9] Studies have shown that clinical outcomes after alteplase therapy are time-dependent.[10] This urgency of treatment, when coupled with the shortage of onsite stroke expertise, contributes to difficulties for rural and underresourced hospitals to deliver alteplase in a timely manner. Telestroke promotes the safe and reliable administration of alteplase at these remote locations, resulting in a significant increase in the rates of alteplase utilization and shorter door-to-needle times before access to telestroke services.[4,8,11]

Telestroke utilization is linked to improved functional outcomes in the treatment of acute ischemic stroke. Patients who receive intravenous alteplase within 90 minutes of symptom onset are more than three times likely to experience favorable outcomes than patients who did not receive alteplase.[9] Additionally, patients treated with intravenous alteplase at a comprehensive stroke center showed no difference in functional outcomes at 90 days or in discharge outcome and treatment complications when compared with patients who received alteplase at community hospitals via telestroke.[5]

In addition to being among the leading causes of death, stroke also leads to physical and cognitive impairments that impact functional abilities and quality of life. Prompt identification, emergency response, and acute treatment and management of early stroke symptoms impact clinical outcomes. Telestroke has emerged as an important resource to ensure timely access to stroke neurology specialists fostering acute stroke diagnosis and treatment recommendations, recognition of stroke cause and risk, and provision of tools for health promotion strategies for stroke prevention.[7]

It is challenging to quantify quality of life, but the quality-adjusted life-year has been used as a measure to assess the value for cost of a health care intervention. A 2013 model to estimate the incremental costs and effectiveness of a telestroke network found that when compared with no network, a telestroke network yielded a discounted cost savings of $1000 to $1900 per patient and an incremental effectiveness of 0.01 to 0.03 quality-adjusted life-years per patient.[12] These results illustrate the health care resource utilization savings and cost-effective benefits from a societal perspective caused by improved clinical outcomes ameliorated by telestroke.

BARRIERS TO USE OF TELESTROKE

Despite the overall benefit of telestroke utilization, many barriers (eg, **Box 2**) exist that may limit stroke hospital participation in a telestroke network. Common challenges related to licensure and liability include infrastructure funding, regulatory changes to promote the development of acute stroke–capable or primary stroke centers, reimbursement for services, physician adoption and participation, licensure and credentialing issues, technology assessment and deployment, medical liability, compliance with privacy laws, and compliance with fraud and abuse statutes.[4] Under the telestroke model, the on-site treating physician and the remote consulting physician need to be licensed to practice medicine in the state where the patient is located, and both providers must be credentialed and privileged at the originating site. For a telestroke hub serving multiple spokes, consulting neurologists must be credentialed at all spoke hospitals in the network. This process is time-consuming and cumbersome, requiring significant administrative resources to ensure that all credentialing requirements are met. This process is more limiting when the spoke hospital is in a different state than the hub. Under the traditional state-based physician licensure system, each state requires that physicians practicing medicine in the state are licensed by that state. Telemedicine advocates are lobbying for relaxing the methods of telemedicine licensure by instituting reciprocity between states or developing a national licensure system.[6]

Widespread use of telemedicine is hindered by limitations in reimbursement; legal issues, such as state licensure laws; the need for multiple-site credentialing; and liability concerns. Insurance coverage for telehealth is fragmented: only 29 states (double the number for 3 years ago) have telehealth parity laws that require private insurers to cover telehealth services to the same extent that they cover in-person care.[7] There exist 48 state Medicaid programs, each with its own restrictions, that cover telehealth services. Medicare only reimburses telemedicine services to clinical facilities in areas where there is a shortage of health professionals.[13] Potential solutions to these limitations include the accelerated implementation of the Interstate Medical Licensure Compact and the Tele-Med Act of 2015, which enable Medicare-participating providers to provide services to any Medicare beneficiary; streamlining the credentialing process at spoke sites by allowing reliance on privileging decisions at hub sites; and providing informed consent to stroke patients regarding telemedicine.[4]

Telestroke reimbursement must also comply with two federal statutes, the Antikickback Statute and the Stark Law, which determine the allowable relationship between hospitals and the sharing of information technology. These statutes prohibit reimbursement for services in exchange for referrals that are payable under programs such as Medicare and Medicaid. This prohibits the hub hospital from providing services or equipment at less than fair market value in exchange for patient referrals to the hub.[4]

Box 2
Barriers to telestroke utilization

Reimbursement

Licensure and liability laws

Technological

Financial

Compliance

The technology necessary for telestroke services poses a challenge to spoke hospitals seeking to engage and sustain membership in a telestroke network. Inadequate training and needlessly complex and sophisticated equipment diminish the efficacy of telemedicine. Technical problems, such as nonconnection, poor broadband access, and malfunctioning devices, are major barriers to successful telestroke programs. The necessity of cloud-based imaging transfer can also cause technological difficulties leading to low levels of satisfaction by hub and spoke. This can delay care, especially in spoke facilities that lack immediate image interpretation by a radiologist. The lack of interoperability between computer systems and between electronic medical records may delay adoption of telestroke because of the rapid obsolescence of technology and potentially wasted capital.[4]

Financial barriers to telestroke utilization exist on the hub and spoke side. Spoke hospitals must invest in the purchase and maintenance of computer hardware and software; they need to maintain a secure way to transmit stroke-related data that is compliant with federal privacy standards. Hub hospitals must recruit and provide round-the-clock access to vascular neurologists while also providing training and support for spoke hospital clinical staff. The lack of adequate reimbursement to physicians and hospitals has played a crucial role in delaying the development of sufficient acute stroke call coverage, which may profoundly affect smaller, nonacademic hospitals.[4] A surprising financial barrier to telestroke is the reimbursement policy for "drip and ship," a term referring to cases in which thrombolytic therapy is initiated at the spoke hospital during a telestroke consultation, and then the patient is transferred to a comprehensive stroke center, typically the hub hospital, for the remainder of treatment. In this drip-and-ship scenario, Medicare does not permit either the spoke or hub hospital to obtain enhanced payment, even if alteplase is still infusing on arrival to the hub hospital; rather, the spoke hospital is only paid on an outpatient basis for the medication, and the receiving hospital is only paid the traditional inpatient payment rate for stroke care of patients not receiving thrombolytic therapy.[5] A final financial barrier is the lack of resources a spoke hospital may experience providing postacute stroke care for patients not transferred to the hub hospital, with or without thrombolytic therapy.[11]

REDUCING COSTS WITH TELESTROKE

Research suggests that telestroke utilization can be cost-effective, can improve continuity of care, can shorten hospital stays, avoid unnecessary transfers, enhance education, and improve research trial enrollment.[4] Although telestroke has an upfront implementation cost, its utilization can lead to reduced health care costs, direct and indirect, by reducing acute care lengths of stay and long-term care needs.[5] It is clear that when considering the overall lifetime costs of managing patients impacted by stroke, reducing or eliminating complications and disability results in health care resource savings.[8] It has been estimated that the use of remote patient monitoring for certain patients with chronic conditions could yield $1.8 billion in savings over 10 years.[10]

Telestroke also contributes to cost reduction by reducing complications and disabilities by initiating timely cost-effective interventions at the point of care, such as intravenous alteplase, or by identifying and facilitating patient transfer to higher levels of care for specific interventions, such as neurointensive care, decompressive hemicraniectomy for life-threatening cerebral infarction with swelling, and emergent surgical or endovascular repair of ruptured aneurysms and mechanical thrombectomy.[4]

The overall lifetime costs of managing stroke is estimated to be $62.7 billion annually in the United States, with a 15% to 30% rate of permanent disability and 20% of stroke victims requiring institutional care 3 months post-stroke.[4] The national increase in intravenous alteplase administration rates because of telestroke has been estimated to avoid direct costs of $13.6 million, reduce acute care days by 4351, reduce residential care days by 43,902, and save $5.2 million in indirect costs annually.[5] Telestroke can provide better access to post-stroke care. Newer applications of telestroke include virtual rehabilitation therapies, offering patients the opportunity to participate in physical and occupational therapist-supervised therapies closer to their homes and support systems, eliminating long transfers and reducing family travel costs.[5]

NURSES ROLE IN TELESTROKE

The stroke delivery model at the spoke hospital is greatly impacted by telestroke utilization. Nurses at the spoke level become coordinators of acute stroke care. Several elements of nursing care include triage in the emergency department, care of the patient including vital signs, intravenous access, blood work, timely computed tomography scan arrival, blood pressure evaluation and management, neurologic assessment using the National Institutes of Health Stroke Scale, documentation of a stroke code, and administration of intravenous alteplase.[14] Depending on the spoke hospital policy, nurses may be responsible for calculating the alteplase dose; mixing the medication; administering a bolus; starting the infusion; and monitoring the patient receiving alteplase for complications, such as angioedema and hemorrhagic transformation.[14] Improving the scope, quality, and speed of stroke treatment requires nurse leaders to create a structure for a spoke hospital's stroke care delivery model.

SUMMARY

Stroke is a leading cause of disability and death in the United States in the adult population. Telestroke can provide increasing access to expert stroke care and treatment that promote quality outcomes and reduce costs in stroke care. It provides an effective solution for providing underresourced hospitals access to acute stroke expertise. With access to stroke experts, stroke disability and death could decrease.

Many quality outcomes are achieved with the use of telestroke. It can increase the access to acute stroke care, thereby providing timely assessment, accurate diagnosis, and effective treatment. Telestroke has been linked to improve functional outcomes in the treatment of acute ischemic strokes.

There are currently several barriers to providing a telestroke service. Common challenges include: licensure and liability, reimbursement, technology, and financial issues. It is important to recognize these barriers and begin to implement strategies to overcome these barriers.

Telestroke engages nurses at the spoke hospital to become coordinators of acute stroke care, which identifies the need and avenues for educational and professional development.

Telestroke utilization can be cost-effective. It can reduce complications and disabilities by initiating timely interventions. The future of telestroke is beginning to provide improved access to post-stroke care.

REFERENCES

1. Centers for Disease Control and Prevention. Stroke. 2018. Available at: https://www.cdc.gov/stroke/index.htm. Accessed December 19, 2018.

2. LaMonte M, Bahouth M, Xiao Y, et al. Outcomes from a comprehensive stroke telemedicine program. Telemed J E Health 2008;4:339–44.

3. Burch S, Gray D, Sharp J. The power and potential of telehealth what health systems should know: proposed legislation in Congress offers the promise that the nation's healthcare policy will support the expansion of telehealth, allowing hospitals and health systems to fully realize the benefits of this important emerging approach to care. Healthc Financ Manage 2017;2:46–50.

4. Dorsey E, Topol E. State of telehealth. N Engl J Med 2016;2:154–61.

5. Kulcsar M, Gilchrist S, George M. Improving stroke outcomes in rural areas through telestroke programs: an examination of barriers, facilitators, and state policies. Telemed J E Health 2014;1:3–10.

6. Bowen P. Early identification, rapid response, and effective treatment of acute stroke: utilizing teleneurology to ensure optimal clinical outcomes. Medsurg Nurs 2016;4:241.

7. Adler-Milstein J, Kvedar J, Bates D. Telehealth among US hospitals: several factors, including state reimbursement and licensure policies, influence adoption. Health Aff 2014;2:207–15.

8. Demaerschalk B, Berg J, Chong B, et al. American Telemedicine Association: telestroke guidelines. Telemed J E Health 2017;5:376–89.

9. Almallouhi E, Holmstedt CA, Harvey J, et al. Long-term functional outcome of telestroke patients treated under drip-and-stay paradigm compared with patients treated in a comprehensive stroke center: a single center experience. Telemed J E Health 2018. https://doi.org/10.1089/tmj.2018.0137.

10. Al Kasab S, Harvey J, Debenham E, et al. Door to needle time over telestroke: a comprehensive stroke center experience. Telemed J E Health 2018;2:111–5.

11. Baratloo A, Rahimpour L, Abushouk A, et al. Effects of telestroke on thrombolysis times and outcomes: a meta-analysis. Prehosp Emerg Care 2018;22(4):472–84.

12. Demaerschalk B, Switzer J, Xie J, et al. Cost utility of hub-and-spoke telestroke networks from societal perspective. Am J Manag Care 2013;12:976–85.

13. Amorim E, Shih M, Koehler S, et al. Impact of telemedicine implementation in thrombolytic use for acute ischemic stroke: the University of Pittsburgh Medical Center telestroke network experience. J Stroke Cerebrovasc Dis 2013;4:527–31.

14. Rafter R, Kelly T. Nursing implementation of a telestroke programme in a community hospital in the US. J Nurs Manag 2011;19:193–200.

Impact of a Mobility Team on Intensive Care Unit Patient Outcomes

Jennifer Ratcliffe, DNP, MSN, RN[a],[*],[1], Brandy Williams, MSN, RN[b],[1]

KEYWORDS

- Critical care • Intensive care • Mobility physical therapy • Mobility team
- ICU liberation

KEY POINTS

- Mobility of ICU patients improves long-term outcomes.
- Although clinical practice guidelines are in place and benefits of mobility are well documented, a culture of immobility prevails in many ICUs.
- Challenges in mobilizing ICU patients can include lack of therapy staff and consultations.
- Use of a dedicated mobility team can increase number of patients mobilized, empower nursing staff, and improve patient outcomes.

INTRODUCTION

In recent years, there has been an escalation of peer-reviewed publications, research teams, and implementation of quality initiatives around the nation and the world that reflect the prioritization of improving patient outcomes after an intensive care unit (ICU) stay. Critical illness is often catabolic and debilitating, and many survivors experience residual effects that affect long-term physical functionality and quality of life.[1] ICU-acquired muscle weakness frequently occurs in this patient population and is strongly associated with the culture of immobility and bed rest that has historically been present in ICU settings[2]

Early mobilization of critically ill patients in the ICU setting has been shown to improve long- and short-term outcomes[3] and has been demonstrated to be safe and attainable[4] and profoundly beneficial.[5] Significant evidence documents the benefits of early mobilization in ICU settings to include[6,7]:

- Decreased hospital and ICU length of stay
- Decreased duration of mechanical ventilation

[a] Patient Care and Quality; [b] Cardiac and Critical Care Services
[1] 4500 13th Street, Gulfport, MS 39501.
* Corresponding author.
E-mail address: joratcliffe@mhg.com

Crit Care Nurs Clin N Am 31 (2019) 141–151
https://doi.org/10.1016/j.cnc.2019.02.002
0899-5885/19/© 2019 Elsevier Inc. All rights reserved.

ccnursing.theclinics.com

- Greater ambulation distance
- Better functional outcomes at hospital discharge

Implementation of an early mobility program, however, can present numerous challenges[8] In many facilities, it represents a paradigm shift in the treatment of critically ill patients because ICU patients may remain immobilized for prolonged intervals[9] or even the entire duration of time when receiving mechanical ventilation.[10] Achieving a culture of early mobility is also heavily influenced by issues and variability in staffing patterns and resources available for early intervention activities.[11]

BACKGROUND

Memorial Hospital at Gulfport is a not-for-profit community hospital with 303 beds, a level II trauma center, and two ICUs. The ICU functions as one unit in terms of management and staffing, but in two separate and distinct locations within the facility. One of the ICUs supports a cardiac and cardiac surgery patient population, and the other ICU supports neurologic and medical patient populations. There are 26 total ICU beds split between the two locations supported by a staff of approximately 100 registered nurses (including full-time, part-time, and prn employees). Additionally, five intensivist physicians and six acute care nurse practitioners provide 24-hour (in person) coverage and are available at the bedside any time the nursing staff requires provider assistance along the trajectory of patient care.

In October of 2015, the ICU leadership team began meeting in an effort to implement the Society of Critical Care Medicine's 2013 Clinical Practice Guidelines for Pain, Agitation and Delirium by using the ABCDEF bundle.[12] At the time, none of the bundle elements were used in practice, and a 3-year plan was drafted to guide change and implement each element of the bundle separately. A culture of oversedation and immobilization prevailed, and the physical therapy (PT) and occupational therapy (OT) staff worked with only 38.4% of the ICU patient population. Moreover, therapy staffing allotments for the ICU setting were limited. This, coupled with a lack of consultations for PT/OT from the provider group caused in part by a lack of prioritization for mobility and an ICU culture that was not aggressive with mobility accounted for the low percentage of patients receiving therapy or mobilization on a regular basis. Additionally, nursing staff expressed apprehension regarding the safety of mobilizing critically ill patients because they believed there was a lack of multiskilled technicians (MSTs) to assist with turning, lack of PT/OT presence in the unit, and underutilization of the mobilization equipment available. To address this situation, an ICU liberation initiative including the formation of an ICU mobility team was approved to serve as a catalyst for changing the culture of immobility in the ICU setting, and to empower the team to provide care with the goal of improving long- and short-term outcomes for critically ill patients.

PROPOSED OUTCOMES OF MOBILITY TEAM

The long-term outcomes of creating a mobility team were to meet the early mobility element (E) of the ABCEDF bundles and create a culture of mobility within the ICUs without an increase in cost to the institution. In addition to meeting the E element, other long-term goals were to meet the element without an increase in the ICU patient fall rate.

PLANNING

Although the implementation of the early mobility and exercise component (E) of the ABCDEF bundle was one of the last elements to be implemented in practice, it was perhaps the most positively accepted component in this bundle of evidence-based care.[13] The ICU mobility team was formed and consisted of staff members that were placed in MST positions to allow for a broad scope of the position. This facilitated collaboration with all members of the interprofessional team (physicians, ICU nurses, nurse practitioners, and therapy staff) and provided autonomy for mobilizing patients.

The ICU staff enthusiastically welcomed the mobility team and supported their valuable addition and contribution to the interprofessional team. The recruitment of these team members occurred in-house and included staff that were previously employed in transporter and various technician positions that required patient contact on many and varied units (including ICU) and some limited assistance with patient mobility. Thus, the new mobility team staff were knowledgeable about transporting patients, familiar with patient positioning, and comfortable in the ICU environment.

Orientation began with classes for MSTs on the mobility team offered by the professional development department to include training for documentation in the electronic health care record (EHR); back safety and patient positioning in-services; and training on safe management of catheters, use of patient lift devices, and safe patient handling. On completion of these classes, MSTs job shadowed with PT and OT staff to establish familiarity with workflow and patient load and advanced training in functional mobility and use of assistive devices. Job shadowing also occurred with ICU nurses for familiarization and safe practice with a wide variety of tubing, lines, and devices commonly used in the ICU patient population. The mobility team also received in-depth in-services on patient positioning by the wound care nursing staff. This training included proper positioning to offset pressure on the bony prominences, side-to-side position changes, repositioning to avoid shearing injuries, and optimal positioning to prevent patient being too close to side rails. Demonstration of techniques, such as floating extremities at the proper angle, proper techniques for bending knees, and correct technique for floating arms and heels were also used. The wound care nursing staff also highlighted having empathy for patients that are unable to reposition themselves and an in-depth discussion on awareness of all bony prominences.

Orientation to use of the bedside monitoring systems, ICU specialty beds, safe handling of ventilated patients, and the supine cycle equipment were also provided. The supine cycle was purchased for the ICU in early 2016 to assist with implementation of the E bundle for the ICU mobility team initiative. Before formation of the mobility team, the supine cycle was not used since purchase. The portable supine cycle is used with patients confined to the bed and allows them to participate in physical activity while spending time in bed immobilized or tethered to lifesaving mechanical systems. The supine cycle is mounted on an adjustable table that slides over the patient bed for use and provides several activity modes to accommodate fluctuations in ICU patient participation.

This structured orientation occurred over approximately a 4-week period with ongoing updates and refreshers provided as needed.

Data Collection and Analysis

The Acute Physiology and Chronic Health Evaluation (APACHE) tool was used for data collection and outcomes measurement during the implementation of the ICU liberation project. APACHE is a tool that serves as an adjunct to the EHR and provides clinicians with decision support and performance management. The APACHE system includes risk-adjusted outcome measures, built-in and ad hoc reporting capabilities, and comparative reporting solutions. APACHE data were analyzed using descriptive statistics. Additionally, a performance improvement analyst was used to aggregate and interpret data outcomes.

IMPLEMENTATION

In December of 2016, the ICU mobility team was formally operationalized and staffed in both ICUs Monday to Friday. This team of five MSTs became responsible for assisting the PT/OT staff in meeting patient needs with direct supervision provided by the acute therapy manager (a physical therapist) that also supervises all acute PT, OT, and speech therapy staff. The ICU bedside nurse was tasked with direct communication with the mobility team about the patient's status, assistance with mobility, and assessment of tolerance of mobility activities.

Daily Workflow

The ICU mobility team consists of five MSTs that work in collaboration with physical therapists and occupational therapists (**Fig. 1**). Two of the MSTs on the team are assigned to each ICU Monday through Friday from 0630 to 1415. On arrival to their work area, a chart review is conducted of each ICU patient. Patients are individually assessed for mobility appropriateness in collaboration with PT/OT by using the facility's provider-approved list of exclusion criteria for ICU mobilization (**Box 1**).

The ICU mobility team coordinates with ICU nursing staff to establish a plan of care and workflow for each individual patient. The mobility team identifies patients that have planned procedures and new patients in the ICU, and adapts to unexpected changes that occur during their workday. The PT/OT team prioritizes ICU patient consultations and evaluations early in their shift to better collaborate and integrate care with the ICU mobility team, and the team assists PT/OT with mobility during their evaluations as needed. The team also communicates with the acute therapy manager regularly during their work day to provide updates.

Patients are assisted with functional mobility throughout the shift by the mobility team to include such activities as toileting, meal assistance, sitting, standing, and

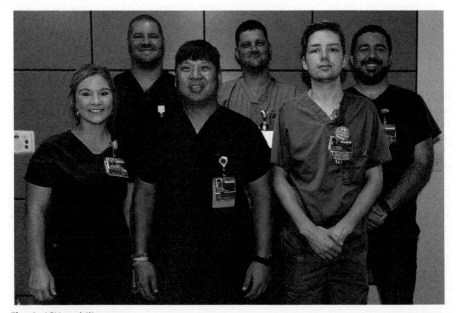

Fig. 1. ICU mobility team.

Box 1
Exclusion criteria for ICU mobilization

- Active bleeding
- Active myocardial infarction
- Arctic Sun (targeted temperature management) in use
- Arterial/venous sheath
- Comfort care measures
- Cordis in groin
- External ventriculostomy drain or ICP bolt device*
- Femoral arterial line?
- F_{Io2} greater than 60% and/or PEEP greater than 8
- Hemodialysis catheter in groin
- Hemodynamically unstable requiring more than one vasoactive medication
- IABP or Impella device in place
- Leg or pelvic fractures (activity, PT/OT per orthopedics)
- Lumbar drain
- Open abdomen or chest incision
- Paralytic agent in use
- Position restrictions ordered
- Spinal precautions (activity, PT/OT per orthopedics)
- TPA administration within the last 24 hours
- Tracheostomy placement within 24 hours
- Traction excluding Halo

Abbreviations: F_{Io2}, fraction of inspired oxygen; ICP, intracranial pressure; PEEP, positive end-expiratory pressure; TPA, tissue plasminogen activator.

---

ambulation. Postoperative mobility orders for surgical patients are implemented by the mobility team, and passive range of motion exercises are performed on patients that meet exclusion criteria for mobility or are otherwise unable to be mobilized. All documentation of activities of daily living completed with each ICU patient is recorded in the EHR by team members.

Additionally, the mobility team is responsible for turning all ICU patients every 2 hours by using the ICU turn clock (**Fig. 2**), and for keeping all ICU patients on a consistent turn schedule. The team advocated for elimination of the supine position on the ICU turn clock during an ICU quality improvement hospital-acquired pressure injury (HAPI) initiative and the suggestion was approved and implemented in both ICUs. The team voiced that ICU patients are often placed in the supine position for bedside procedures, such as line placement, chest radiograph, dialysis, bronchoscopies, and meals, and could remain in the supine position for more time than desirable. The mobility team believed that by eliminating supine position, it would prevent excess time on their backs and potentially prevent skin breakdown. Documentation of turning in the EHR also became the responsibility of the mobility team with nursing oversight.

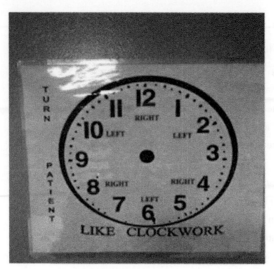

Fig. 2. Turn clock.

In addition to assistance with functional mobility and activities of daily living, responsibility for the weight accuracy and proper usage of the ICU specialty beds was assumed by the mobility team. The mobility team assesses each patient's skin integrity with all mobility encounters, and concerns or alterations in skin integrity are immediately reported to PT/OT and nursing staff. The ICU mobility team also assists the ICU coordinators when performing weekly skin assessments for HAPI prevention.

To help ensure a continued culture of mobility when the ICU mobility team and/or PT/OT staff are not present on the unit, daily usage of the laminated ICU mobility cards was implemented (**Fig. 3**). These communication tools assist in the continuum of mobility care and awareness between shift and staff changes. After PT/OT and/or provider approval, the cards are marked to indicate the patient's designated level of mobility for the oncoming shift. After the implementation of the mobility team, they assumed responsibility for updating and usage of the cards, which were rarely or inconsistently used since their creation early in 2016. Suggestions for a user-friendly design were proposed by the team and the existing cards were edited to make the change. Increased usage of mobility cards encouraged mobilization activities when PT/OT staff were not physically present, and bolstered the confidence and comfort level of the night shift nursing staff to mobilize their patients at the appropriate level.

After formation of the mobility team, the daily workflow also included assessment of appropriateness of the supine cycle (in collaboration with the PT/OT staff) with patients placed on the supine cycle when suitable. Consequently, usage of the supine cycle went from zero to approximately 10%.

Other responsibilities of the mobility team include daily assistance with patient mobility activities on the progressive care unit when needed and daily and weekly data collection to track patient outcomes. Mobility team members are rotated between ICUs on a 6-month basis to promote flexibility and familiarity with the two ICU environments and the various ICU health care team members.

OUTCOMES OF MOBILITY TEAM
Patient Outcomes

As a result of the initiation of a mobility team, PT/OT consultations for ICU patients increased from 38.4% (n = 915) in 2016 to 78.1% (n = 1862) in 2017, and then to

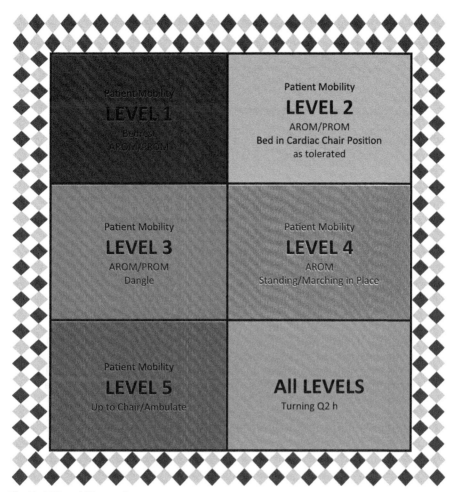

Fig. 3. ICU mobility cards.

86.2% (n = 1382) for first through third quarters in 2018. ICU length of stay (**Fig. 4**) had a statistically significant downward trend (n = 6435). The ICU length of stay before implementation of the mobility team was 3.06 days and dropped to 2.41 days and is currently (3Q18) at 2.57 days, demonstrating a significant downward trend. Furthermore, ICU readmissions (**Fig. 5**) also showed a downward trend (n = 422). The ICU readmission rate before implementation of the mobility team was 6.8% and trended as low as 3.5%. An increase in the readmission rate was noted in 3Q18 and will be monitored. Although this trend was not statistically significant, it was better than predicted values from the APACHE scoring system. Ventilator days had a slight (**Fig. 6**) decrease overall but not statistically significant. Total actual number of patients on the ventilator on Day 1 in ICU were 1146 in 2016, 1126 in 2017, and 833 in first quarter through third quarter 2018.

The total number of patients in the ICU that were ambulated had a percentage increase of 80% from 2016 to third quarter of 2018. In 2016, 7.8% of ICU patients (n = 187) were ambulated in the ICU, and in quarters one to three of 2018, 14% of ICU patients (n = 234) ambulated while in the ICU. The ambulation distance in feet

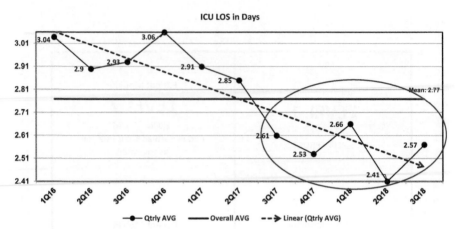

Fig. 4. ICU length of stay.

has also pointedly increased (**Fig. 7**). Additionally, the number of patients assisted to a standing position increased from 0.17% (n = 4) in 2016 to 5.1% (n = 122) in 2017, and then 4.7% (n = 78) in first through third quarters of 2018. The percentage of patients receiving passive range of motion went from 58.3% (n = 1390) in 2016 to 60.3% (n = 1438) in 2017, and 67.5% (n = 1125) in first through third quarters of 2018. The percentage dangled on the edge of the bed also increased from 2.27% (n = 54) in 2016 to 10.8% (n = 258) in 2017, and 10% (n = 167) in quarters one through three in 2018 (**Fig. 8**). Also of note, before the implementation of the mobility team and ICU adoption of ABCDEF bundle, no ventilated patients in the ICU were mobilized.

There was no significant increase in adverse events in ICU patients noted since the implementation of the mobility team in December of 2016 through the third quarter of 2018. Fall rates have remained unchanged and at baseline, and hospital inpatient quality reporting system events revealed no fall occurrences related to mobility team activities. We did not see a significant change in the ICU HAPI rate during this timeframe.

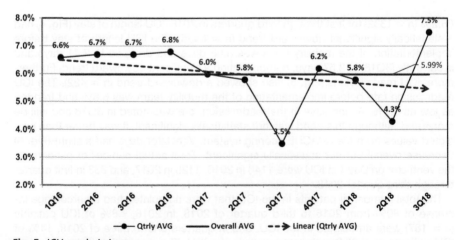

Fig. 5. ICU readmissions.

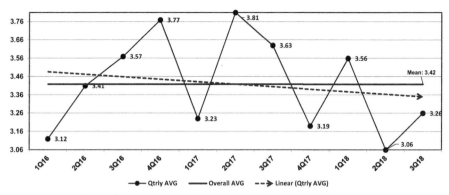

Fig. 6. ICU ventilator days.

Staff Outcomes

A survey of ICU nurses used pre-implementation and post-implementation of the mobility team was performed. Results indicated that pre-implementation of the mobility team, nursing staff believed the patients were being turned every 2 hours, but did not believe the patients were out of bed as often as clinically appropriate because of a lack of time and support. Post-implementation results revealed that nurses believed turning was still a priority and agreed that patients were out of bed any time they meet appropriate criteria (did not meet exclusion criteria). Nursing staff believed they had more time and were well supported with mobilization of patients. Concerns related to patient safety and self-injury were also improved. The nursing staff surveyed strongly agreed that the addition of the mobility team increased overall nurse satisfaction and believed that mobility team staffing should be expanded to include night and weekend coverage.

Cost Outcomes

The financial impact of implementation of a dedicated mobility team resulted in positive outcomes in relation to ICU staff injures. Since inception of the mobility team in December 2016, there have been no ICU staff injuries related to patient handling. This number represents a significant decrease from the 2 years before implementation when five injuries occurred in 2015 and 2016 (**Fig. 9**).

DISCUSSION

The implementation of a mobility team in the ICU was successful in meeting the E element bundle of the ICU liberation initiative. It proved to be a cost-effective way

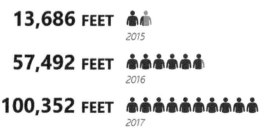

Fig. 7. Distance of ambulation.

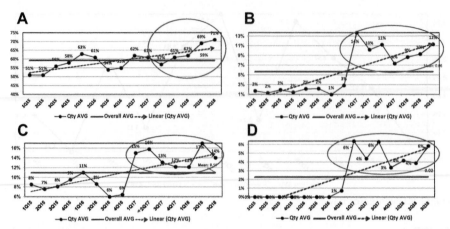

Fig. 8. Activity summary run charts. (*A*) Percentage of ICU patients receiving range of motion (ROM). Data points 3Q17–3Q18 show an upward trend for percentage of patients receiving range of motion in the ICU. (*B*) Percentage of ICU patients dangled. (*C*) Percentage of ICU patients ambulated. (*D*) Percentage of ICU patients standing.

to meet the early mobility element without a substantial increase in cost and offsetting the use of costly PT units. Implementation and training were fairly simple processes, and nursing staff felt more supported and open to mobilizing critically ill patients. The culture of immobility in the ICU setting shifted to one that viewed mobility as medicine with a more positive and enthusiastic response to PT and OT presence and participation in the continuum of patient care.

SUMMARY

Early mobility in the ICU may minimize loss of functional abilities and thereby shorten hospital stays. Use of a dedicated mobility team in the ICU setting demands a collaborative approach among members of the multidisciplinary team to coordinate care and provide safe mobilization of patients. Patient and cost outcomes of the impact

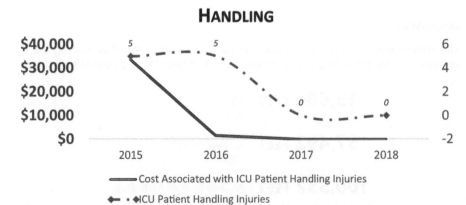

Fig. 9. ICU patient handling. ANOVA, analysis of variance; LC; UC.

of a mobility team at Memorial Hospital in Gulfport will continue to be monitored, tracked, and trended quarterly to assess effectiveness of the team long-term, and recommendations for expansion into night and weekend coverage and coverage in the progressive care unit are currently being discussed.

REFERENCES

1. Hermans G, Van Mechelen H, Clerckx B, et al. Acute outcomes and 1-year mortality of intensive care unit–acquired weakness. A cohort study and propensity-matched analysis. Am J Respir Crit Care Med 2014;190:410–20.
2. Dinglas VD, Aronson Friedman L, Colantuoni E, et al. Muscle weakness and 5-year survival in acute respiratory distress syndrome survivors. Crit Care Med 2017;45:446–53.
3. Cameron S, Ball I, Cepinskas G, et al. Early mobilization in the critical care unit: a review of adult and pediatric literature. J Crit Care 2015;30(4):664–72.
4. Dubb R, Nydahl P, Hermes C, et al. Barriers and strategies for early mobilization of patients in intensive care units. Ann Am Thorac Soc 2016;13(5):724–30.
5. Adler J, Malone D. Early mobilization in the intensive care unit: a systematic review. Cardiopulm Phys Ther J 2012;23:5–13.
6. Danmeyer J, Dickinson S, Packard D, et al. Building a protocol to guide mobility in the ICU. Crit Care Nurs Q 2013;36(1):37–49.
7. Needham DM, Wozniak AW, Hough CL, et al, National Institutes of Health NHLBI ARDS Network. Risk factors for physical impairment after acute lung injury in a national, multicenter study. Am J Respir Crit Care Med 2014;189:1214–24.
8. Rose B, Forry C. Integrating a mobility champion in the intensive care unit. Dimens Crit Care Nurs 2018;37(4):201–9.
9. Brower RG. Consequences of bed rest. Crit Care Med 2009;37(10 Suppl): S422–8.
10. Mendez-Tellez PA, Nusr R, Feldman D, et al. Early physical rehabilitation in the ICU: a review for the neurohospitalist. Neurohospitalist 2012;2(3):96–105.
11. Fraser D, Spiva L, Forman W, et al. Original research: implementation of an early mobility program in an ICU. Am J Nurs 2015;115(12):49–58.
12. Barr J, Fraser GL, Puntillo K, et al. Clinical practice guidelines for the management of pain, agitation, and delirium in adult patients in the intensive care unit. Crit Care Med 2013;41:263–306.
13. Devlin JW, Skrobik Y, Gelinas C, et al. Clinical practice guidelines for the prevention and management of pain, agitation/sedation, delirium, immobility, and sleep disruption in adult patients in the ICU. Crit Care Med 2018;46(9):e825–73.

Leadership's Impact on Quality, Outcomes, and Costs

Linda Roussel, PhD, RN, CNL*

KEYWORDS

- Mindfulness leadership • Creativity • Curiosity • Uncertainty • Safety • Efficiency

KEY POINTS

- A mindfulness leader uses communication, relationship-building, and situational awareness strategies to model attention to surroundings in space and time. Paying attention, being aware, and increased sensitivity to others can alert one to possible safety breaches and danger ahead, thus mitigating risk for avoidable error. Mindfulness leadership also improves value-based outcomes, including reduced patient and employee costs.
- A mindfulness leader is a role model through exquisite communication and collaboration skills, asking great questions, and coaching through humble inquiry. Team members are encouraged to think out loud and share ideas, thoughts, and perspectives, thus increasing the idea pool for greater sharing and collaboration.
- A mindfulness leader engages team members in so-called what if and plus thinking, which can be playful and productive, and is critical to advancing outcomes and to improving patient and employee outcomes in complex dynamic health care settings.

INTRODUCTION

Leadership is being influential and modeling the way. Kouzes and Posner[1] describe a leaders' ability to break down bureaucracy, particularly when it stifles curious, creative thinking. Leaders model an action orientation, trying new and different ways of approaching improvement for better outcomes. Mindfulness leaders can read the signposts and see the 30,000-foot view when team members are hesitant about where to go and how to get there. Mindfulness leaders cocreate opportunities for small successes along the way, providing ways to further improve and excel in meeting organizational systems' quality outcomes. Efficiency and effectiveness in providing safe, quality care are not a matter of either-or; both are essential to a sustained effect.

Disclosure Statement: The author has nothing to disclose.
Texas Woman's University, College of Nursing, ASB 129, P.O. Box 425498, Denton, TX 76204, USA
* 1415 Denise Drive, New Braunfels, TX 78130.
E-mail address: lroussel@twu.edu

Having influence can have an impact on quality care, patient safety, and effective and efficient systems.[2] Improvement and quality work are enhanced by leaders who create a culture of innovation in which a fail-fast system is encouraged and safe. Codesigning work spaces that stimulate all the senses requires that mindful leaders be intentional in their every thought and action in leading people and systems. Leadership in the allocation of resources (time, attention, feedback, listening), removing barriers, and facilitating meaningful conversations are great places to start.[3] High-tech firms, such as China's innovative digital giant, Alibaba, have gone far to streamline operations, increasing efficiencies in routine work processes and dazzling end users' experiences.[4] According to Campbell,[4] "digital leaders no longer manage; rather, they enable workers to innovate and facilitate the core feedback loop of user responses to firm decisions and execution." He goes on to describe the leader's mandate to cultivate creativity to increase innovation uptake as efficient systems are being built into daily operations. By leading efforts to create a culture of curiosity and creativity, innovation readily happens and thrives. Innovation can become the order of the day and woven into the day-to-day fabric of work experiences by careful execution of resources, particularly talent and ingenuity. This article explores mindfulness leadership practices by making the business case for creativity and curiosity, as well as their links to quality, outcomes, and effective and efficient systems.

DESIGN THINKING

Design thinking can enhance new ways of working in chaotic and uncertain times. Working through the steps in design thinking facilitates mindful leaders' innovations by focusing on empathy, defining with greater clarity and focus, ideation, prototyping, and testing.[5] Design thinking involves discovering the customer experience through immersion, sense-making, and alignment. Creating ideas through immersion and articulation, leaders have a desire for movement through the testing experience, both before the experience and while learning in action. "Recognizing organizations as collections of human beings who are motivated by varying perspectives and emotions, design thinking emphasizes management, dialogue, and learning. That is social technology at work."[5]

Design thinking promotes exploring uncertainty for improved collaboration and better outcomes. Uncertainty motivates leaders to find better ways to improve quality, outcomes, and efficiency. Mindful leaders increase awareness of facilitators and barriers to a curious environment by being inquisitive, welcoming feedback and insights, and supporting creative work spaces. Leaders can model the way by appreciating the art of asking great questions in the face of uncertainty and encouraging others in appreciating best practices in having meaningful conversations. Mindfulness leadership integrates creativity and curiosity during times of uncertainty. Qualities of mindfulness, as described by Kabat-Zinn,[6] include attitudes such as trust, patience, gratitude, acceptance, not judging, and generosity. Ellen Langer,[7] a prominent Harvard researcher on mindfulness, illuminates the role of awareness of our surroundings. As Langer[7] shares, "mindfulness is the very simple process of actively noticing new things. When you actively notice new things, that puts you in the present, makes you sensitive to context. As you are noticing new things, it is engaging, and it turns out, after a lot of research, that we find that it is literally, not just figuratively, enlivening."[7] **Fig. 1** illustrates how mindfulness leadership characteristics can integrate key concepts of creativity and curiosity in a time of great uncertainty. As the leader notices surroundings, creates context, and shares observations, emotional intelligence and exquisite communication skills can only enhance the influence and impact on organizational systems' outcomes.

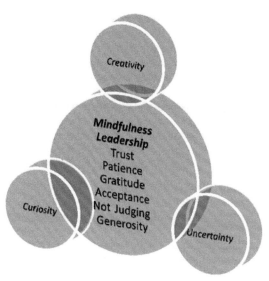

Fig. 1. Mindfulness leadership.

It is not enough to measure outcomes; appreciating the process of getting there provides better and more efficient ways to innovate for improvement. Constant communication and collaboration; for example, the Toyota 5 whys strategy, reinforces continuous improvement through questioning.[8] Mindfulness leaders practice awareness and ongoing reflection of their thinking and action orientation.

MINDFULNESS LEADERSHIP, IMPROVED COMMUNICATION, AND BEING CURIOUS

In her Technology, Entertainment, Design (TED) Talk, Headlee[9] provides 10 ways to have a better conversation. She shares excellent strategies that can enhance communication and confidence in bringing out the best in teams and interpersonal relationships. Improvement depends on a team's ability to share ideas and collaborate effectively. Having 1 great conversation at a time can go far toward that end. The 10 basic tips Headlee[9] shares for having great conversations follow:

1. Listening. This is the most important strategy. If you listen wholeheartedly, this alone can yield amazing outcomes.
2. Be honest about what you do not know. If you do not know, say that you do not know. You are perceived as more authentic and trustworthy if you are truthful about how and what you communicate in an honest and sincere way.
3. Use open-ended questions. Guiding questions that ask for greater clarity, exploration, and inquiry can readily establish rapport and an interest in what the other person is sharing. This can lead to greater insights, increasing the pool of information and wisdom of the team.
4. Not sweating the details. Headlee[9] shares that it is important to "stay out of the weeds" because struggling to find exact dates, times, and unimportant details can be distracting and takes away from the flow of the conversation.
5. Not multitasking. Be present and really be there. If you cannot be present, it is best to get out of the conversation. Checking your phone (or other digital devices) can be distracting and inhibits your ability to follow the flow of the communication, often requiring you to repeat information, and fragments the conversation.

6. Appreciate the other person's experience. Your experience is your experience. Be open to what the other person is saying because their experience is personal and unique. You want to know your team members' perspectives, and interrupting to share your personal experience can be disrespectful and dismissing.
7. Be brief. This means sharing (when it's your turn to share) in a succinct, meaningful way with clarity and focus.
8. Everyone is an expert in something. Be curious and open to learning new information. Approach every conversation with a spirit of inquiry and curiosity.
9. Try not to repeat yourself. Headlee[9] considers this condescending and boring.
10. Go with the flow. This can happen naturally if you are really listening to the other person, and want to understand what is being communicated.

Covey,[10] in *The 7 Habits of Highly Effective People*, describes the importance of first seeking to understand. This creates opportunity for the person you are communicating with to share his or her true self, providing insights that you may never hear if you are trying to force impressions. Be prepared to be amazed.

Being curious and asking great questions opens up others to being willing to dig deeper and perhaps share more. Increasing the reservoir of new ideas, different ways of thinking, unimaginable insights, can only improve innovation. Without creating a culture of curiosity, it is unlikely that new ways of being and doing in the organization will occur. Being curious and encouraging creativity through mindful leadership and design thinking, particularly in uncertain and chaotic times, can open new channels for information flow and innovation.

Gino,[11] in the *Harvard Business Review* article "The Business Case for Curiosity," describes the benefits of curiosity, highlighting the essential nature of improving positive outcomes and facilitating healthier work environments. Gino[11] shares that fewer decision-making errors, more innovation, and positive changes in creative and noncreative jobs, reduced group conflict. She notes that more open communication and better team performance are specific benefits of creating a culture of curiosity, stating "When we are curious, we view situations more creatively and have fewer defensive reactions to stress." Gino[11] shared that, in groups that encourage curiosity about their projects, team members tend to put themselves in another's shoes and take an interest in another's ideas rather than focusing only on their own ideas. This creates greater communication and collaboration, something we all are striving for in our work and project teams. Being curious can enhance the health care improvement leader's skills in setting a vision and establishing goals. Structure need not compromise curious and creative work.

CREATING A COMMON VISION FOR GREATER EFFICIENCY: CURIOSITY MATTERS

Understanding the need to establish a common vision and compelling realistic (and stretch) goals are keys to engaging stakeholders. A vision is essential for contextualizing the future. Once this is established, leaders must communicate the vision to those involved in executing the mission and goals. Carrying out the mission and goals for quality care can be hindered if barriers to building a curious, creative culture are not addressed. Specifically, leaders may find it difficult to let go as staff members explore different ways of engaging patients, families, and team members. It may be difficult for managers to challenge standard operating procedures, particularly if current systems seem to be running smoothly. We may want business as usual because our routines may seem to reduce uncertainty and anxiety if we are confident in executing our daily work. Why be disruptive when our work is good enough and we are meeting our metrics, measures, and dashboard outcomes? The mindfulness leader is comfortable with uncertainty and disruption, particularly when they lead toward innovation and continuous improvement. Being comfortable with ambiguity and mindful that process improvement takes time as part of the iterative cycle of change can provide a sense of peace and appreciation for growth and development along the way. Being uncomfortable with uncertainty may thwart questioning because leaders may seek efficiency at the detriment of exploration.

Value-based purchasing and being good financial stewards may seem at odds with organizational cultures that support inquiring minds, curiosity, and innovation. We need not think either-or but instead embrace a perspective of and-both as being efficient, effective, exploratory, and inquisitive. Martin[12] provides a theoretic underpinning for integrative thinking to consider and-both scenarios. Specifically, Martin[12] offers 4 stages of decision-making from an integrative thinking perspective:

1. Determining salience. Integrative thinkers embrace the messiness of life and complexity. They resist a limited number of solutions, and consider both sides of the argument or the decision to be made.
2. Analyzing causality. Considering alternatives and options affords a multiple perspective of problem-solving versus a singular, linear cause-and-effect course of action. Using salient solutions from the first step of integrative thinking provides more options to thoughtfully ponder.
3. Envisioning the decision architecture. According to Martin,[12] "Integrative thinkers don't break down a problem into independent pieces and work on them separately or in a certain order. They see the entire architecture of the problem—how the various parts of it fit together, how one decision will affect another. Just as important, they hold all of those pieces suspended in their minds at once."[12]
4. Achieving resolution. Working through the steps provides opportunities for considering several solutions and perspectives. Although it may be challenging to get to this point, mindfulness leaders welcome integrative thinking and model these best practices for team members.

Integrative thinkers create cultures that demonstrate creativity, curiosity, and innovation, and flourish within their organizational systems. This must be done with intention and steadfast pursuit, pushing team members to go beyond the status quo and business as usual. This is particularly challenging for health care leaders because they often face life and death issues, and are concerned about going out on a limb to innovate steady systems.

BEST PRACTICES IN CREATING A CULTURE OF CURIOSITY

In "The Business Case for Curiosity," Gino[11] describes 5 ways to bolster curiosity:

1. Hire for curiosity. Google and IDEO are examples of companies that look for intellectually curious individuals.
2. Model inquisitiveness. As a leader, asking great questions, resisting judgment, and truly practicing listening can provide real-time modeling and nurture exploration and discovery. "Experience and expertise exacerbate the problem: As people climb the ladder, they think they have less to learn. Leaders also tend to believe they're expected to talk and provide answers, not ask questions."[11]
3. Emphasize learning goals. Leaders can stress the importance of learning and goal-setting happening in tandem, as well as using mediocre goals as a springboard to better ones. Gino[11] describes Pixar's technique of plussing, which is the building on ideas without using judgmental language. For example, a starting point might be, "I like our current approach to transitioning our patients from the intensive

care unit to the medical unit, and what if we …?" The idea is for another team member to jump in with another plus. This technique may be considered a type of brainstorming, adding an element of inquisitiveness to team learning. "This technique allows team members to remain curious, listen actively, respect the opinions of others, and contribute their own."[11] This process embraces sharing of all types of ideas to be investigated, with leaders broadcasting a clear message that learning is an essential goal even if it does not lead to success. Opening up ways to share in safe, fun, and inviting ways can lead to new ideas and innovations. Staats,[13] in *Never Stop Learning*, describes ways to create learning organizations. Leaders can facilitate learning by modeling ways to learn from failure, focus on process, ask the right questions, recharge and reflect, be ones' true self, play to strengths, make today special, seek variety tomorrow, and learn from others. His strategies are further illustrated through wonderful stories and narratives that provide exemplars to test ways organizations can create a culture of inquiring and ongoing learning.

4. Let employees explore and broaden their interests. Although an organization may not be able to provide free time for employees to work on their own projects, there can be opportunities for cross-pollination by teams. For example, using design thinking principles, ideation as a step in the process may involve nursing, engineering, information technology, and marketing. Although nursing may take the lead in the team's collaboration, it is the skills each member brings, and the questions asked and the ideas explored, that broadens the perspective. Prototypes can be designed based on the diversity of ideas from the various world views of each member. There is often an appreciation of each other's skills and a sense of holism when coming together. The author had the opportunity to work with biomedical engineering faculty and students while teaching and immersing clinical nurse leader (CNL) students during their clinical rotation. Using design thinking principles and working alongside biomedical engineering students, the CNL students were able to extend their understanding of the microsystem's gaps and needs, providing new ways to deliver safe, effective care. This underscores patient-centered care and paying attention to the patient's experience, which we are all struggling to address, and provides greater real-time innovation and flow.

5. Have Why? What if? How might we? days. Using the Toyota 5 whys approach can change the mindset of team members toward innovation and challenge existing perspectives.

The future of a business' success lies in the ability of leaders to foster an environment in which creativity is the order of the day. Campbell,[4] in his article "Alibaba and the Future of Business," shared lessons from China's innovative digital giant, describing advancement from the use of big data management, algorithms, deep learning, and machine learning. Specifically, he states that in the "smart business model, machine learning algorithms take on much of the burden of incremental improvement making adjustments that increase systemwide efficiency." With more efficient systems in place, the leader's most important role is to foster creativity and increase the success rate of innovation, rather than to improve the efficiency of the operation. Creativity and innovation are important to patient safety and to a culture of greater effectiveness and efficiency.

LEADING CHANGE FOR EFFECTIVE AND EFFICIENT HEALTH CARE SYSTEMS

As health care providers, the importance of leading change is underscored by our outcomes not proving as positive as we would like. Ellner,[14] vice chair of surgery and director of surgical quality at Saint Francis Hospital and Medical Center in Hartford,

Connecticut, directed a patient safety initiative that reduced the operating room's infection rates by 75%.[14] He shares the 5 dimensions of leadership he believes are required to gain success in a patient safety initiative:

1. Alignment. Ellner[14] purports that identifying change champions is important to providing role models for teaching others about change. Introducing new initiatives is a leader's initial work, before passing them on to those team who are pushing to make changes.
2. Self-awareness. Leading a patient safety project and changing a culture necessitates mindfulness leadership, self-awareness, and empowerment of the team. Working from their strengths, leaders need to understand their own motives and style when inspiring others to act. With an action orientation, leaders do more than outline necessary steps (particularly without input from team members) to drive improvement. Removing barriers and facilitating the use of evidence-based tools presents the leader as a source of influence, particularly in stressful times. Listening to others, and ensuring meaningful conversations improves awareness for all involved.
3. Team-building. We have learned much from research on team science, particularly about wanting all members to participate from their strengths and seeking opportunities for improvement. Creating a team charter and an action plan are included in the process. Working in teams only happens when the organization's culture expects that employees will work together. Trust, communication, relationship-building, and being one's authentic self are expectations that the mindful leader makes transparent in the organization. Not being afraid of speaking up about near misses or adverse events is a hallmark of a trusting culture. Fear of retaliation creates unnecessary stress and anxiety, which can be allayed through creation of a caring and nurturing environment.
4. Leading up. Mindfulness leadership aligns with giving team members opportunities to develop and grow professionally. Leading with the courage of one's convictions can provide powerful modeling for future team success. Effective communication and meaningful conversations are skills necessary to leading up.
5. Leading across. Working with front-line workers and those transforming care at the point of care are essential to patient safety outcomes. Listening for messages, getting and giving feedback, and sharing insights are important in messaging initiatives.

These 5 dimensions provide additional strategies for leading to improve patient safety initiatives and gaining support from leaders across the organizational spectrum for sustainable changes.[14]

Another resource when considering leadership strategies to improve quality patient outcomes within effective and efficient organizations comes from the work of Institute of Healthcare Improvement (IHI) in creating the IHI Leadership Alliance.[15] Specifically, the Alliance is a collaborative endeavor of health system executives and teams who align the goals of working together in partnering with patients, workforces, and communities with the philosophy of fulfilling the promise of the IHI Triple Aim of better health, better care, and lower cost for the populations served. The IHI Alliance has been described as a learning community fostering generosity, curiosity, and courage. The IHI Alliance[15] becomes particularly important as health care systems move from volume-based to value-based systems and as leaders confront new and different challenges that necessitate new ideas, behaviors, and actions. Institute of Healthcare Improvement (IHI) continues to provide innovative strategies and solutions to help leaders at all levels in care delivery organizations find solutions by focusing their leadership efforts in aligning with the Triple Aim (improving patient experience of care, enhancing populations' health, reducing per capita cost of health care) and advancing to the Quadruple Aim (attaining joy in work).

MINDFULNESS LEADERSHIP AND A CULTURE OF IMPROVEMENT

The science of improvement is at the core of the IHI's work of providing useful tools and techniques for sustainable improvement.[8] Specifically, the Model for Improvement (MFI) and collaborative learning through their open school resources assists health care leaders in developing and testing innovative methods when considering small tests of change, using the plan-do-study-act (PDSA) method to sustain and spread positive outcomes. Learning by doing with support of creative, essential resources, can help align learners in health care organizations achieve collective effect. According to the IHI,[8] the MFI "and collaborative learning and improvement anchor our approach to project design and evaluation, implementation, spread, and scale-up in diverse environments and contexts." As an applied science, emphasis is on creative innovative processes, rapid experimentation through in iterative cycle testing in the field, and fostering the spread of learning at all levels. The science of improvement is an applied science that focuses on innovation, rapid-cycle testing in the field, and spread to generate learning about which changes produce improvements. Expert subject knowledge, along with an array of improvement methods and tools, are aligned from a multidisciplinary perspective, drawing from clinical science, systems theory, psychology and behavioral sciences, statistics, and other fields.

As noted by IHI improvement experts, working hand in hand with partners ensures that all improvement efforts include identifying a measurable aim, a measurement framework to support addressing the aim, and delineating the ideas (content) and how these ideas will likely affect the results.[8] Improvement efforts also include outlining an execution strategy to ensure reliable adoption of the content, and doing rapid cycle testing (PDSA) to predict and learn from the iterative cycles. Building on the iterative cycle, leaders use process or value stream maps to provide tangible, concrete steps in the flow of work. Leaders learn from variation and heterogeneity by understanding and using data to determine common or special cause effects for improvement. The leader applies behavioral and social sciences to better understand the theory of change, and to influence outcomes through effective mindfulness leadership. The author's work with CNL and nursing administrative (NA) students illustrates the extensive use of resources from the IHI, particularly the MFI and the use of PDSA cycles. Both student programs (CNL, NA) expected students to do impactful projects using methodological frameworks, metrics, and other tools offered by IHI. Reducing pressure ulcer rates, initiating pet therapy in an acute care setting, and improving follow-up and reducing readmissions for patients with heart failure are but a few examples of projects implemented to improve outcomes. The CNL and NA students, immersed in their microsystems and macrosystems, completed a gap analysis, created a team charter, and used tools such as failure model effect analysis and root cause analysis to collaborate with their interdisciplinary teams when identifying metrics that matter. The use of resources and references provided a common language and methods that facilitated improved communication and collaboration.[8]

MINDFULNESS LEADERSHIP AND SAFETY

Mindfulness goes beyond a person's thoughts and emotions. We know the dangers of going on autopilot, which puts everyone at risk for missing cues of danger ahead. Situational awareness improves when we practice mindfulness in the workplace. Situational awareness can be described as the perception of elements in the environment in a volume of time and space, understanding their meaning, and projecting their status in the future.[16] Three defining attributes of situational awareness include perception, comprehension, and projection. Situational awareness is essential for maintaining a safety culture. Teaching breathing techniques and body scan strategies can improve situational awareness. We know that a person who is situationally aware pays attention to their environments and relationships in their work and personal spaces. Situational awareness includes remaining attuned to a multitude of stimuli, such as bodily sensations, and the ways those sensations influence movement through space, time, and interactions with others. We likely have noted individuals reading their cell phones while walking, not paying attention to their environment, who end up tripping, falling, and injuring themselves.[16] Orique and Despins[17] report that the Occupational Safety Health Administration identifies the 4 top hazards for construction fatalities, including struck by visible objects in the worksite, wandering into unsafe (preventable) situations, falls, and electrocution, which have been tied to concerns related to focus and awareness. Research underscores that workers who are inattentive to their surroundings are more likely to experience an incident. Mindfulness leadership promotes coaching and modeling ways for employees to increase their situational awareness, which is key to safe and quality outcomes in the workplace, and to a quality lifestyle.[17]

MINDFULNESS LEADERSHIP AND EFFECTIVENESS

Mindfulness leadership can have a powerful impact on improving effective and efficient health care by promoting a gentler, kinder culture. Gelles,[18] in *Mindful Work: How Meditation is Changing Business from the Inside Out*, describes mindfulness going mainstream in a variety of companies, including Google, Aetna, General Mills, and Target. All these companies have fostered mindful practice among their workers. A University of North Carolina (UNC) Chapel Hill Kenan-Flagler Business School study[19] reports that the benefits of mindfulness are improved innovative thinking and communication skills, and more timely reactions to stress. These benefits are important in promoting leading-edge and dynamic work, as well as improving day-to-day efficiency. For example, Aetna reports lower health care costs as a result of mindfulness training. Specifically, Aetna partnered with the American Viniyoga Institute and eMindful to do a small pilot program with 239 employees.[18] The results revealed that participants in the 12-week courses (either gentle yoga focused on stress-reduction or a Mindfulness at Work program by eMindful) reported significant stress reduction. Stress in the workplace adds greater, often hidden, costs. Stress costs American businesses an estimated $300 billion annually.[18] It has also been suggested that the costs to the health care system would be higher given the role stress plays in conditions such as heart disease, high blood pressure, and diabetes. Additional findings from the Aetna pilot revealed that more than one-quarter of Aetna's work force of 50,000 had participated in at least 1 mindfulness class, and those who have reported, on average, a 28% reduction in their stress levels, a 20% improvement in sleep quality, and a 19% reduction in pain.[18] Also reported were greater effectiveness on the job and the gain of an average of 62 minutes per week of productivity, each of which Aetna estimates is worth $3000 per employee per year. Aetna also described that the annual health care costs of employees who participated in the program were an average of $2000 lower than their counterparts.[18] Given these stunning gains, Aetna, the health care giant, expanded the program significantly to include a full one-third of its employees.[18] Another example of mindfulness leadership and its impact on an efficient workplace comes from Intel. An early adopter of mindfulness,

Intel began its Awake@Intel program in 2012.[19] Specifically, 1500 employees who participated in a 19-sesson course ranked their level of stress and happiness on a 10-point scale. At the end of the sessions, participating employees described their average levels of stress decreasing by 2 points and levels of happiness increasing by 3 points.[19] Improving joy in the workplace also translated into having new ideas, insights, mental clarity, creativity, and ability to focus; better quality of work relationships; and increased level of engagement in meetings, projects, and team efforts. Although findings were self-reports and difficult to quantify, Intel found the results significantly promising and expanded the program to more than 10,000 employees.[19]

SUMMARY

As we move forward to increase our effectiveness in valued-based organizational cultures, we are charged as mindfulness leaders to innovate by creating environments that foster curiosity and creativity in our uncertain times. Being mindful can increase situational awareness and improve communication, enhancing a culture of safety and better patient outcomes. Mindfulness leadership matters and it provides more effective ways to communicate and collaborate with others. Results matter and increasing our ability to sustain improvement through better awareness can enhance healthy work environments and joy in the workplace.

REFERENCES

1. Kouzes J, Posner B. The leadership challenge: achieve the extraordinary. Available at: http://www.leadershipchallenge.com/about-section-our approach.aspx. Accessed December 12, 2018.
2. Mosadeghrad AM. Factors influencing healthcare service quality. Int J Health Policy Manag 2014;3(2):77–89.
3. Jordan EF, Lanham HJ, Crabtree BJ, et al. The role of conversation in health care interventions: enabling sensemaking and learning. Implement Sci 2009;4:15. Available at: https://implementationscience.biomedcentral.com/articles/10.1186/1748-5908-4-15. Accessed December 12, 2018.
4. Campbell H. Alibaba and the future of business, Lessons from China's innovative digital giant. Harvard Business Review 2018;88–96.
5. Liedtka J. Why design thinking works. Harvard Business Review 2018;72–9.
6. Kabat-Zinn J. The way of mediation: nine attitudes to deepen mindfulness. Available at: https://www.thewayofmeditation.com.au/blog/9-attitudes deepen mindfulness. Accessed December 12, 2018.
7. Langer E. Science of mindlessness and mindfulness.. Available at: https://onbeing.org/programs/ellen-langer-science-of-mindlessness-and mindfulness-nov2017/. Accessed December 12, 2018.
8. Institute for Healthcare Improvement. The science of improvement. Available at: http://www.ihi.org/about/Pages/ScienceofImprovement.aspx. Accessed December 12, 2018.
9. Headlee C. Ten ways to have a better conversation. TedTalk; 2015. Available at: https://www.ted.com/talks/celeste_headlee_10_ways_to_have_a_better_conveation?language=en. Accessed December 12, 2018.
10. Covey S. The 7 habits of highly effective people. New York: Free Press; 1989.
11. Gino F. The business case for curiosity. Harvard Business Review; 2018. p. 48–57.

12. Martin RL. How successful leaders think. 2007. Harvard Business Review. Available at: https://hbr.org/2007/06/how-successful-leaders-think. Accessed December 12, 2018.
13. Staats BR. Never stop learning: stay relevant, reinvent yourself, and thrive. Boston (MA): Harvard Business Review Press; 2018.
14. Ellner S. 5 leadership dimensions needed for patient safety initiatives 2013. Available at: https://www.beckershospitalreview.com/quality/5 leadership-dimensions-needed-for-patient-safety-initiatives.html. Accessed December 12, 2018.
15. Institute for Healthcare Improvement. IHI leadership alliance. Available at: http://www.ihi.org/Engage/collaboratives/LeadershipAlliance/Pages/default.aspx17. Accessed December 12, 2018.
16. Wilbert L. Safety and situational awareness: staying present and focused 2016. Available at: https://www.beaconohss.com/blog/safety-and-situational-awareness-staying-present-and-focused/. Accessed December 12, 2018.
17. Orique D, Despins L. Evaluating situation awareness: an integrative review. West J Nurs Res 2018;40(3):388–424.
18. Gelles D. Mindful work: how meditation is changing business from the inside out. New York: Houghton Mifflin Harcourt; 2015.
19. Schaufenbuel K. Bringing mindfulness to the workplace 2014. Available at: https://www.kenan-flagler.unc.edu/~/media/Files/documents/executive-development/unc-white-paper-bringing-mindfulness-to-the-workplace_final.pdf. UNC Kenan-Flagler Business School Executive Development. Accessed December 12, 2018.

Health Care Information Technology
Moving from Support to Performing Care

Bennett Cheramie, MSN, RN, CHCiO*

KEYWORDS

- Health care • IT • Health technology • Electronic medical record • EMR
- Data analytics • Meaningful use • MIPS

KEY POINTS

- Technology in health care has spanned several decades. Over the last 60 years, technology has grown to be part of all health care. Technology initially transformed the business office and moved to the clinical space capturing data.
- HiMSS EMRAM developed a roadmap to move hospitals and healthcare into the electronic world. The Federal Government developed aided in adoption with the development of the Meaningful Use (MU) program. With a roadmap and a incentive mechanism Electronic Medical Records (EMR) grew from 20% to 100% in under 10 years.
- The Centers for Medicare Services (CMS), since its inception, has attempted to create alternative payment structures that compensate health care providers for quality care. EMR's aid in the measurement of quality, giving rise to the need for Healthcare Analytics and the need for Interoperability amongst different EMR platforms.

TECHNOLOGY RISING IN HEALTH CARE

Technology has been a part of health care as early as the 1960s. The initial technology components drove process efficiencies around automating manual logging, aiding in the streamlining of back office processes.[1] The design of electronic medical records (EMRs) can be tracked back to the late 1960s and 1970s. From this inception, technology has grown and permeated all lifecycles in health care. There are several milestones that have catalyzed the health care information technology (IT) movement. Each milestone created a moment whereby technology would create process efficiencies, improve quality, and control expense. Each milestone is important, but the ultimate goal of health care technology today is to aid in the collection and measurement of data. The medical field and health care in general have always been a data-driven industry.[2] This article will cover how technology has evolved and the milestones along the journey to today, where technology has woven itself into the fabric of the health care industry.

General Health System, Baton Rouge, LA, USA
* 8490 Picardy Avenue, Suite 400, Baton Rouge, LA 70809, USA.
E-mail address: Bennett.cheramie@brgeneral.org

Crit Care Nurs Clin N Am 31 (2019) 165–176
https://doi.org/10.1016/j.cnc.2019.02.004
0899-5885/19/© 2019 Elsevier Inc. All rights reserved.

ccnursing.theclinics.com

In the late 1980s, the development of database structures, particularly "hierarchical or relational" databases were created for health care.[1] These databases laid the foundation for the collection and storage of health care data. The first clinical EMRs were developed and used on these foundational structures in the 1980s. These databases were originally created to streamline billing and collections, and back office processing. The high cost of the hardware at the time made the use of these early EMRs outside of academic settings nearly impossible. It was not until the development of micro-computing in the late 1980s and early 1990s that the hardware became affordable for health care entities other than academics. In addition, the early 1990s gave society the use of personal computing, the Internet, and the ability to set up "networking" between multiple computers that made technology affordable and efficient in all industries including health care.[1]

TECHNOLOGY LANGUAGE DEVELOPMENT

In the early 1990s, along with the collection of demographic data for billing, IT began to scan images into Picture Archiving and Communication Systems (PACS). These systems allowed health care to connect demographic data with clinical data. Along with PACS, other standard exchange terminology emerged, such as Systematized Nomenclature of Medicine – Clinical Terms and Logical Observation Identifiers Names and Codes and the American Society for Testing Materials. The connection and movement of messages or data points from one system to another required these systems to not simply store standard data in a standard way but rather "speak a language." Health Level Seven (HL7) was born as the language that most health care technology software(s) used to communicate within itself and with other systems.[1] HL7 was first created in the 1970s, but the real growth was from 1987 to 1992, when HL7 became the standard language for health care software. HL7 in 1992 "became the most practical solution to aggregate ancillary systems like laboratory, microbiology, electrocardiogram, echocardiography, and other results into a central EMR."[1(pp48–50)] There have been several interactions of HL7, but it remains the standard today.[3]

The early 1990s can be defined as the beginning of the EMR movement, with all innovations available to health care. Health care entities began to see value in the ability to combine clinical documentation with billing/demographic information and the connection between payer and hospital became digitalized. In the late 1990s and early 2000s, EMRs were being created by large academic institutions. "A 2004 Random Sample of health care facilities from across the United States found that 13% of respondents had an EMR system fully implemented while 10% did not have or did not plan to have an EMR system. Most respondents (62%) used a vendor EMR system."[1(pS51)]

QUALITY AND TECHNOLOGY

EMR growth was fueled in the early 1990s by the quality movement when the Institute of Medicine published *To Err is Human*. This publication estimates that 98,000 people die in any given year from medical errors that happen in hospitals. *To Err is Human* asserts that health care is riddled with flawed processes that should be streamlined to improve the quality of care provided in hospitals.[4] The EMR became a vehicle to help streamline clinical processes and a potential solution to improve quality in health care.

In the early 2000s, along with the push from the Institute of Medicine, there were several technologies that were installed from billing, imaging, laboratory, radiology, pharmacy, clinical orders, nursing documentation, and physician documentation.[4]

Each of these were complex and considered to improve both efficiency and quality on 4 fronts: (1) automation, (2) reduction of interpretation, (3) standardization, and (4) ability to measure. Ancillary systems automated many manual checks and balances (eg, pharmacy processing of medications in hospitals). Handwritten orders and documentation required human interpretation, whereas Computerized Order Entry created a standard language and removed the need to interrupt hand writing. Lastly, with EMRs, health care data can be reviewed real-time instead of through manual abstraction and data sampling to aggregate data. Health care quality departments could now use real-time data instead of 3- to 6-month lag times in data aggregation.

THE BIG LEAP

The question becomes, how do we do change from a paper to an electronic system? To help answer this question, in 2005 the Healthcare Information Management Systems Society (HiMSS) developed the HiMSS Electronic Medical Record Adoption Model (HiMSS EMRAM), as illustrated in **Fig. 1**. EMRAM created a roadmap for health care to implement systems and the order in which they should adopt these systems. More importantly, it outlined how hospitals could cascade change with health care IT in an order that supported a hierarchical approach to implementation of supporting operations. The model outlines a 7-stage approach to adopting health care technology that systems worldwide could use to stage implementation. The model outlined installing foundational systems such as registration and ancillary systems in stage 1 and higher level processes, for example, full clinical decision support (CDS), at stage 7.

EMR and health care technology in the mid 2000s now had a value proposition, and a playbook for hospitals on how and why to install such systems. These technology initiatives remain complex and costly for hospitals and health care organizations.

HEALTH INFORMATION TECHNOLOGY FOR ECONOMIC AND CLINICAL HEALTH AND MEANINGFUL USE PROGRAM

In 2008, The Office of the National Coordinator for Healthcare Technology (ONC) passed legislation to stimulate the growth and adoption of EMRs. The Health Information Technology for Economic and Clinical Health (HITECH) Act of 2009 outlined the Meaningful Use (MU) program. This program provided economic stimulus for health care entities that adopted EMRs. The program also created penalties for organizations that did not adopt an EMR in the mandated time period. Meaningful Use outlined criteria or outcomes that defined what a "Meaningful User" of health care technology had to measure and achieve as part of annual MU application. Meaningful Use criteria was amended from year to year and both the number and baseline achievement metrics increased. For example, year 1 measures had to be started and show a minimal compliance percentage, but year 4 of the same measure required 100% compliance. Meaningful Use mandated that EMR technology must also be certified by the ONC for hospitals to enroll in the MU program. Through the annual certification process, the ONC was able to provide direction to EMR vendors on what to develop within the software to meet the growing regulatory demands around quality outcome measures. The mandate for Certified Electronic Healthcare Record Technology (CEHRT) standards for MU eligibility among EMR vendors, essentially obsoleted self-developed or home-grown EMR. This process, in which the ONC drives software development through EMR certification to meet the needs of the regulatory agencies (eg, Centers for Medicare Services or CMS) was born during the MU timeframe (2008–2015) and persists today.

STAGE	HiMSS Analytics EMRAM EMR Adoption Model Cumulative Capabilities
7	Complete EMR; External HIE; Data Analytics, Governance, Disaster Recovery, Privacy and Security
6	Technology Enabled Medication, Blood Products, and Human Milk Administration; Risk Reporting; Full CDS
5	Physician documentation using structured templates; Intrusion/Device Protection
4	CPOE with CDS; Nursing and Allied Health Documentation; Basic Business Continuity
3	Nursing and Allied Health Documentation; eMAR; Role-Based Security
2	CDR; Internal Interoperability; Basic Security
1	Ancillaries - Laboratory, Pharmacy, and Radiology/Cardiology information systems; PACS; Digital non-DICOM image management
0	All three ancillaries not installed

Fig. 1. EMR adoption model cumulative capabilities. (*From* HiMSS Analytics. himssanalytics.org. Electronic medical record adoption model. 2018. Available at: https://www.himssanalytics.org/emram. Accessed October 2, 2018; with permission.)

Implementation and maintenance of an EMR is a costly undertaking for any health care entity, with the bulk of the expense occurring in the first 3 years of an EMR implementation. That being said, the MU program was designed to address the financial burden during the implementation time frame. During the first 4 years of MU a subsidy is provided for participating hospitals to offset the cost for implementing an EMR. To achieve MU the organization applying for the program must meet criteria, and use a CEHRT EMR; if all criteria are met then the organization receives a government subsidy for that year. This subsidy required yearly application and was only available during the first 4 years of application. If the organization failed to achieve MU in the first 4 years, it lost that year's subsidy, without penalty. In the second 4 years of the 8-year program, the penalty phase was introduced. During the second 4 years of MU and in 2012 hospitals not enrolled in the program or failed to meet the defined measures received a penalty based on a percentage of Medicare reimbursement. The penalty phase included increasing penalties for each year that MU was not achieved up to a maximum of 4% of all Medicare reimbursement. Since Medicare reimbursement is relative to each organization, it affected small and large organizations. The subsidy or carrot helped pay for some EMR cost, but the penalties placed heavy burdens on health care, making MU a "must" do. Adoption Rates of EMR, with associated health care technologies, increased from 10% in 2008 to 96% in 2015 (**Fig. 2**).

The ONC was created as part of the HITECH Act and governs the MU program. As with many governmental regulatory bodies, the ONC modified MU as new knowledge of the positives and negatives of the program were unveiled. The measures were adjusted through comment periods on a yearly basis to assure that all parties (eg,

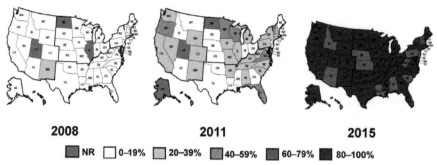

2008   **2011**   **2015**

■ NR   □ 0–19%   ■ 20–39%   ■ 40–59%   ■ 60–79%   ■ 80–100%

Fig. 2. EMR adoption by year. Notes: basic electronic health record (EHR) adoption requires the EHR system to have at least a basic set of EHR functions, including clinician notes, as defined in Table A1. Estimates for states, shaded gray, did not meet the standards for reliability (NR). See Table A2 for a complete list of 2008, 2011, and 2015 hospital adoption by state. (*From* Henry J, Pylypchuk Y, Searcy T, et al. Adoption of electronic health record systems among US non-federal acute care hospitals: 2008–2015. Washington, DC: The Office of National Coordinator for Health Information Technology. Available at: https://www. healthit.gov/sites/default/files/briefs/2015_hospital_adoption_db_v17.pdf; ONC/AHA, AHA Annual Survey Information Technology Supplement.)

vendors, hospitals, clinics) were treated fairly to meet regulations. As adoption grew and MU evolved, there were several elements from using an EMR that can be explored further in the influence of technology and providing care. EMRs provided hospitals and health care with an unlimited supply of data points. Every data element on the continuum of care was now collected. Using an EMR does not in itself improve efficiency. Data collection does not mean data sharing.

With the use of data from EMRs, financial, quality, operational outcome data, etc., were derived by running a few reports rather than weeks, months, and years of manual data abstraction. Using paper document abstraction became obsolete, and health care analytics was now a driver for most hospitals as data were reported and available for interpretation and used to improve patient care. The ability to see "nonstandard" documentation pathways required multiple iterations of process re-engineering making this type of data less available.

OPERATIONAL PROCESS TRUMPS TECHNOLOGY

In early 2010, transformation of clinical workflow included the use of not only a stethoscope but documentation of specific pieces of information into the EMR to allow for measurement. This re-engineered process often created the need for standardization and potential inefficiencies. The EMR, although giving hospitals the ability to measure data, began to cause unease in the medical community, dictating how care was performed and documented, adding "hours" onto a physician's already busy day. From 2010 to 2011, the Chief Medical Information Officer (CMIO) role was adopted by most hospitals, to help manage and keep a balance between efficiency and ability to measure. The CMIO now leads and drives organizational change, often incorporating technology into innovative processes. As a physician, he/she assures that organizations consider process along with function.

BIG DATA

With the evolution of data collection, organizations began to create analytics programs and departments, with massive data warehouses and visualization software.

Hospitals, payers, and multiple software vendors developed datasets and created data isolations on how care quality could be improved by driving best practice through data. The ability to prove decision support fits in the HiMSS analytics EMRAM model, and the MU regulation, which made analytics or big data something everybody wanted. In 2013, Dan Ariely, Professor of Psychology and Behavioral Economics, tweeted "Big Data is like teenage sex: everyone talks about it, nobody really knows how to do it, everyone thinks that everyone else is doing it, therefore I want to do it."[5]

"Big Data" needs to have big value. The definition of big data remains somewhat fuzzy, but includes data analysis, hypothesis generation, and not testing.[6] Big data or analytics often includes data mining, with classification, clustering, and regression.[6] Analytics can combine many data elements to provide physicians and clinicians with CDS systems (CDSS). A simple example is around blood pressure and medication administration. A medication can be flagged by the EMR to measure blood pressure before administration, and can alert the clinician to not give medication if blood pressure is not in range. This example, although simple, can now be a measure as an avoided error in the day-to-day care of the patient with a simple CDSS tool that the EMR and analytics made available. These simple systems can become part of a more complex analytics approach around appropriate administration of medications for particular disease processes, then bundled into larger efforts to affect entire populations of health. This affect or ability to predict or use "predictive analytics," is a core tenant of CDSS. In expanding CDSS, data can be used to not only predict but learn how to treat illness. Emerging technologies advance traditional analytics and "learn" how to diagnose. For example, in 2018 researchers leveraged artificial intelligence (AI) to perform deep learning in reading chest radiography, drawing conclusions that AI-diagnosed pneumonia on chest radiography interpretation was better or "just as good" as a radiologists' interpretation. This created controversial discussion on whether or not radiology would become a dying profession.[7] AI and machine learning is becoming the "next big thing" in health care to help manage patients and populations.

POPULATION HEALTH AND INTEROPERABILITY

Managing populations requires interoperability. Patients, do not receive all their care from just one health care provider. Insurance providers (payers) often drive patients to entities to receive care or treatment for a discounted price. This practice provides a lower cost to the payer and, thus, lower patient cost. Through this process data are fragmented or delayed. For example, a patient receives primary care from a group associated with a health care system in which that patient's clinical data resides, inside that health care system's data warehouse. If the patient were to receive a test, procedure, or emergency visit at a different health care system, those datasets reside in a separate data warehouse. Finding ways to make these data warehouses communicate to each other is a simple definition of creating interoperability. Standard languages, as previously discussed, help match laboratory and radiology test results data, but clinical data have many challenges.

The HITECH Act built in interoperability standards identifying standard components of patient identification and clinical data points that must be shared as part of the MU in a staged, roll-out process.[8] As the ONC regulated and modified MU, billions of data points began to be collected, and the importance of connecting multiple EMR instances became apparent. In the latter stages of MU, the ONC adjusted measures to assure that hospitals were not only implementing EMRs for their patient population, but they were building in processes to connect to other EMRs. The connection between different hospitals and EMR vendors is known as the interoperability movement.[9] As patients receive care at multiple locations, the documentation happens in different EMRs, fragmenting the patient's record. This fragmentation causes incomplete records and duplicate care. As the MU program begins to wind down, record fragmentation makes the need for interoperability and having a "complete" record a most important component to carry forward in future legislation.

The Department of Health and Human Services has a critical responsibility to advance the connectivity of electronic health information and interoperability of health information technology.[1,6] The ONC's 10-Year Vision on Interoperable Health IT Infrastructure identified the need to build interoperability of the EMR foundations produced from the MU program.[1–3,6] Much like the adoption of an EMR in the MU era, the next 10 years should demonstrate rapid adoption of interoperable systems. Today, all 50 states have some form of health care information exchange. States require health care entities to report data from EMRs in a standard format to registries; such as immunizations and chronic condition data. "Individuals should be able to exchange health information with providers securely to support their own health."[9] One significant initiative is through "The Blue Button," where individual consumers and patients are able to see some portion of their personal heath record. This effort is supported by many of the payers. All EMRs, as regulated by the HITECH Act, require the ability to transmit data and receive a Continuity of Care Document. This document is a standard format, identified by the ONC, to ensure that a minimum dataset including medications, allergies, surgical/medical history, are created and can be sent and received by all MU participation EMRs.

To continue the journey to fully integrated and interoperable health care records, there needed to be collaboration between federal agencies, payers, vendors, and health networks across all levels, federal and state. It will require compromise and agreement from EMR vendors and not "lock in" one mechanism to exchange health information.[9]

Managing population health requires interoperability at some level. But what is population health, and can it be performed to some degree? Population health is defined as "the responsive, equitable, and integrated system of service delivery, inclusive of health promotion, disease prevention, treatment, rehabilitation, and palliation aimed at improving health by comprehensively addressing the biological, social, and structural determinants of health using a community-centered approach for a defined population."[2–4,9] Using this definition, if you can identify a population and the disease process, then you can manage that population considering a community-centered approach.[10] This approach aligns with the quality movement and aligns with CMS value-based programs.

TECHNOLOGY AND ACCOUNTABLE CARE ORGANIZATIONS

A major theme in the Affordable Care Act is the triple aim. The triple aim includes adopting patient-centered care and population health, partnered with bending the cost curve of health care. Many of the programs to regulate patient care and population health conditions fall under the regulation of CMS. These regulations consist of innovative payment models that support the idea of compensating physicians and hospitals for achieving certain quality goals. The thinking is that by improving quality and reducing the need for health care, the cost of care is decreased.[11]

To participate in advanced quality improvement programs and to take advantage of these innovative payment models, data collection from various clinical data warehouses are needed. To achieve this data sharing or interoperability and align financial incentives, health care organizations began to form partnerships. These partnerships are known as ACOs. In the ACO model provider groups partner and assume risk. This risk can be identified as a shared saving from Medicare if the groups meet cost and quality goals. In this model, the ACO is governed by the partners; therefore, the practice groups hold each other accountable for achieving or not achieving goals. More importantly, the ACO is at risk for not achieving goals.[11]

A major part of every ACO is the information system that aggregates and provides visualizations of clinical and claims data. Identifying "fall outs" is paramount to minimize risk exposure for the ACO. If the information system cannot provide accurate, near real-time data then the ACO will struggle to maintain its solvency. Most ACO vendors work with multiple EMRs and payer data feeds to help the ACO manage populations and gaps in care. Managing a population was discussed earlier, but gaps in care are a part of population management that requires additional definition as it outlines managing a population with a specific condition, and preventing common chronic conditions that are better managed with early detection. An example of a "gap in care" is the need for colorectal screening on turning 50 years of age. Many primary care physicians manage the need for colorectal screening on the patient's next visit. If a patient turns 50 years of age but does not see his/her primary care physician then the patient has a gap in care. These gaps can lead to disease progression without detection causing additional cost to both the patient and payer. ACOs are tasked with managing these gaps to assure that patients at risk either by age, sex, or comorbidity are managed following best practice. Failure to do so would translate to the ACO not receiving any shared savings, since there are no savings. ACO began forming in 2010, "they doubled from 221 to 486 and now exceed 600."[11]

VOLUME TO VALUE

In 2014, the MU era began to wind down; however, the need for interoperability persisted. The growth of ACOs and CMS desire to achieve the triple aim began to formulate a nationwide movement identified as the move to value. The reason for the moniker, "move to value" referred to the shift in compensation models for health care. In health care today, Medicare and payers compensate physicians and health care organizations on the amount of care or number of patients for whom care is provided, known as a "fee for service" model. The more patients who are seen, or the more procedures performed, the more health care organizations are compensated, volume driven. Moving from a volume-driven health care system to a value-driven health care system, in which providing "less care" can be correlated to improving value yields a saving that is shared between payers and health care organizations. Figuring out how to make the transition from volume to value is the tricky part, how do you change the entire compensation structure without bankrupting health care, and causing collapse?

Value-Based Payment Modifier programs are mainstay for CMS and Department of Health and Hospitals (DHH) to regulate to a quality standard. Value-based programs are mainstay for CMS and DHH to regulate to a quality standard. Historically, especially post-MU, CMS is growing the number of measures health care organizations have to meet. The EMR and MU provided CMS with the ability to measure and benchmark health care organizations. CMS relies heavily on benchmarking with a penalty versus a reward approach. As health care organizations are compared against peers, the organizations that rise to the top receive compensation, while those that fall to the bottom receive penalty. Much like MU, quality measures are adjusted and governed with input and comments by participants to adjust measurements to achieve maximum effect. A main component of the CMS quality initiatives were the Physician Quality Reporting System (PQRS) developed by CMS to unify multiple quality initiatives under one umbrella for eligible physicians.[12] Physician Quality Reporting System was the quality program developed to provide benchmarking for physicians against their peers around a specific group of quality metrics, rewarding physicians that outperformed in their peer group. The last program year for PQRS was 2016, giving way to Medicare Access and Children's Health Insurance Program Reauthorization Act (MACRA) to further consolidate and focus CMS quality improvement efforts.[12]

MEDICARE ACCESS AND CHILDREN'S HEALTH INSURANCE PROGRAM REAUTHORIZATION ACT

To stimulate the transition from "Volume to Value," the 2015 Congress passed the Medicare Access and Children's Health Insurance Program Reauthorization Act. With the passing of MACRA, CMS announced hopes to move 90% of fees for service payment model to a "quality of service" or value model. Another part of MACRA addressed the sustainable growth rate (SGR). The SGR was used by CMS to prevent escalating cost a beneficiary could receive in a given year, essentially controlling the amount a Medicare patient could receive in a given year. In 1997, Congress passed a cap on the SGR in an attempt to control cost. Since that time, there have been several legislative patches to prevent the cap. The MACRA repealed SGR and created a funding mechanism tied to a conversion factor in place until 2026.[12]

The MACRA allows health care organization and practicing physicians to participate in one of 2 ways. The 2 pathways are (1) Merit-Based Incentive Payment System (MIPS) or (2) the Alternative Payment Model (APM). The APM is focused on those health care organizations that are participating in an ACO. The APM takes into account health care organizations or physicians that are in value-based contracts that assume "risk." The difference is that not all ACOs will meet the MACRA minimum requirements of assuming risk in a value-based contract. To participate in the APM model, the ACO must assume "more than nominal financial risk for poor quality outcomes." To remain in the APM program, health care organizations must maintain a required percent (%) of revenue derived from the APM. In 2019 the ACO will have to derive 25% of revenue from the APM and ratchet up to 75% in 2026. If a practice falls short of the APM revenue measure it will be subject to MIPS.[12]

MERIT-BASED INCENTIVE PAYMENT SYSTEM

The Merit-Based Incentive Payment System is the model that will apply to most physicians and health care organizations. The MACRA program is slated to reach maturity in 2026 with the MIPS payment adjustments taking effect in January 2019. The performance period for January 2019 will be for calendar year 2017 and will carry a bonus of +4% to a penalty of −4% of Medicare reimbursement. Much like the MU program and the APM, the benefits and penalties are ratcheted up to a total of ±9% of Medicare reimbursement by the year 2026. The MIPS is broken up into 4 categories and will adjust volume or fee for service payments, to performance in each category. Each category is weighted differently. The 4 categories are (1) quality, (2) advancing care information (ACI), (3) clinical practice improvement activities, and (4) resource use (cost of care).[12] The categories are weighted as follows: quality 50%, resource use (cost of care) 10%, clinical practice improvement activities 15%, and ACI 25%. **Fig. 3** displays the MIPS categories.

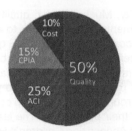

- Quality – Similar to PQRS today
- CPIA – Clinical Improvement activity (ex. care coordination)
- Resource Use – similar to VBPM today
- ACI – Replace MU

Fig. 3. MIPS categories. (*Data from* Jones LK, Raphaelson M, Becker A, et al. MACRA and the future of value-based care. Neurol Clin Pract 2016;6(5):459–65.)

The quality portion is the most heavily weighted for obvious reasons. The CMS had various value-based programs before MACRA. These programs included Hospital-Acquired Condition Reductions, Hospital Readmission Reductions, and Value-Based Purchasing, to name a few. **Fig. 4** displays the timeline for value-based programs. In the CMS 2016 Strategic Plan for Quality, the idea of consolidating all quality initiatives into MACRA and the drive to value-based care was outlined. This move aligns the CMS quality efforts with the legislation and aids to focus strategy around the move to value.[13]

The ACI component of MACRA carries a 25% weight and resembles the MU component. As with MU, ACI is where health care technology fits into the MACRA equation. As mentioned earlier, as the MU program winds down the outstanding need for interoperability persists. Meaningful Use focused on adoption of EMR and advancement of CDS, MACRA, or the ACI component of MACRA focus on promoting and then adopting interoperability.

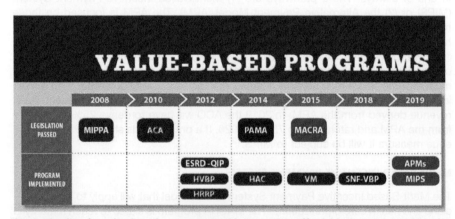

Fig. 4. Timeline for value-based programs. Legislation: ACA, Affordable Care Act; MACRA, the Medicare Access & CHIP Reauthorization Act of 2015; MIPPA, Medicare Improvements for Patients & Providers Act; PAMA, Protecting Access to Medicare Act. Programs: APMs, Alternative Payment Models; ESRD-QIP, End-Stage Renal Disease Quality Incentive program; HACRP, Hospital-Acquired Condition Reduction program; HRRP, Hospital Readmissions Reduction program; HVBP, Hospital Value-Based Purchasing program; MIPS, Merit-Based Incentive Payment System; SNFVBP, Skilled Nursing Facility Value-Based Purchasing program; VM, value modifier or PVBM, physician value-based modifier. (*From* Centers for Medicare & Medicaid Services. Cms.gov. Value-based programs. 2018. Available at: https://www.cms.gov/Medicare/Quality-Initiatives-Patient-Assessment-Instruments/Value-Based-Programs/Value-Based-Programs.html. Accessed October 2, 2018.)

Currently the CMS (year 3) 2018 rule is under review with adjustments to ACI. The current proposed rule overhauls the MIPS ACI category to the Promoting Interoperability category. This restructure is in an effort to create "greater electronic health record interoperability and patient access while aligning with the proposed new Promoting Interoperability Program requirements for hospitals."[14] The rule proposes less objectives and measures and base scoring on Promoting Interoperability, also, care of complex patients, and end-to-end reporting. There are a number of complex patients; there are 4 objective measures with 2 new proposed objectives. The 4 objective measures include e-Prescribing, Health Information Exchange, Provider to Patient Exchange, and Public Health and Clinical Data Exchange. The 2 new objectives include prescription drug monitoring and verify Opioid treatment agreement. All of these objectives are based on a form of interoperability or data exchange. Clinicians are also required to submit some measures electronically and must be using a CEHRT edition EMR to participate on data collecting and reporting. The reporting of metrics across multiple EMRs is an example of end-to-end reporting.[14]

There are several changes to each of the MIPS categories. Adjustments are made to these categories by collecting data from health care entities (eg, hospitals, ACOs, and payers). Participating entities are allowed to provide feedback or comment on the current categories; that data are then collected and analyzed by CMS. There is a 60-day comment period that is now closed. The ability of MACRA to shift the payment model from fee for service to value is yet to be seen. In 2019, the impact on reimbursement and Physician Fee Schedule under MACRA will test if health care can accept the model and adjust practice moving forward.

SUMMARY

Technology in health care has grown in the last 50 years, and exploded in the last 20 years. In today's health care environment, all aspects of care require technology. Health care has seen IT migration from a health care billing system in the 1980s and 1990s to analytics in 2010. We have seen booms in technology adoption with MU and the quality drive. Technology has become part of the fabric of health care. It has been the catalyst for policy and process changes. Technology continues to innovate. With the massive amounts of data collected, the addition of AI and machine learning are invading the health care technology marketplace.

REFERENCES

1. Evans RS. Electronic health records: then, now, and in the future. Yearb Med Inform 2016;20:S48–61.
2. Berenson RA, Rice T. Beyond measurement and reward: methods of motivating quality improvement and accountability. Health Serv Res 2015;50:2155–86.
3. Cowie MR, Blomster JI, Curtis LH, et al. Electronic health records to facilitate clinical research. Clin Res Cardiol 2017;106:1–9.
4. Institute of Medicine. To err is human. Washington, DC: The National Academies Press; 2000.
5. Dan Ariely. 2013. Available at: https://twitter.com/danariely. Accessed January 6, 2013.
6. Lee CH, Yoon HJ. Medical big data: promise and challenges. Kidney Res Clin Pract 2017;36:3–11.
7. Davenpoert TH, Keith J, Dreyer DO. AI will change radiology, but it won't replace radiologists. Harvard Business Review 2018;1–5.

8. Ja Wanna Henry M, Yuriy Pylypchuk P, Talisha Searcy MM, et al. Adoption of electronic health record systems among U.S> Non-Federal acute care hospitals: 2008-2015. Washington, DC: The Office of National Coordinator for Health Informatin Technology; 2016.

9. The Office of National Coordinator for Health Information Technology. A 10- year vision to achieve an interoperable health IT infrastructure. Washington, DC: The Office of National Coordinator for Health Information Technology; 2015.

10. Mercer T, Gardner A, Andama B, et al. Leveraging the power of partnerships: spreading the vision for a population health care delivery model in western Kenya. Global Health 2018;14:44.

11. Ingram R, Scutchfield DF, Costich JF. Public health departments and accountable care organizations: finding common ground in population health. Am J Public Health 2015;105:840–6.

12. Lyell K, Jones JM, Marc Raphaelson M, et al. MACRA and the future of value-based care. Neurol Clin Pract 2016;6:459–65.

13. CMS quality strategy. 2018. CMS.gov CMS Quality Strategy. Retrieved from CMS. gov Centers for Medicare and Medicaid Services. Available at: https://www.cms. gov/Medicare/Quality-Initiatives-Patient-Assessment-Instruments/QualityInitiatives GenInfo/Legacy-Quality-Strategy.html. Accessed September 24, 2018.

14. CMS. Retrieved from quality payment program proposed rule for the quality payment program year 3. 2018. Available at: CMS.gov; https://www.cms.gov/ Medicare/Quality-Payment-Program/Resource-Library/2019-QPP-proposed-rule-fact-sheet.pdf. Accessed September 24, 2018.

Maternal Quality Outcomes and Cost

Cathy Maher-Griffiths, DNS, MSHCM, RN, RNC-OB, NEA-BC*

KEYWORDS

- Maternal morbidity • Maternal mortality • Patient safety bundles
- Perinatal care management • Postpartum hemorrhage
- Hypertensive pregnancy disorders • Maternal sepsis

KEY POINTS

- In the United States, maternal morbidities and mortalities are increasing in contrast to other developed countries. The leading causes of maternal death include cardiovascular diseases, infection and sepsis, and postpartum hemorrhage.
- Evidence-based maternal patient safety bundles and tool kits have not been consistently adopted by hospitals providing obstetric care. There is evidence that the implementation of these bundles and tool kits reduces the incidence of maternal mortality. Maternal mortality reviews, simulation, and essential warning systems provide a framework for achieving improved outcomes.
- Regionalization of maternity care will facilitate the appropriate and timely delivery of maternity care at all levels. Historically, more emphasis has been placed on neonatal levels of care and transport; however, more focus is needed to assure that the mother is in a facility providing the appropriate level of care.
- The operationalization of integrated behavioral health care in the obstetric and gynecologic care settings provides a mechanism for providing a team approach to meet the mother's medical and behavioral health requirements. Preconception care needs to be standardized to improve maternal outcomes.

INTRODUCTION

In the United States over the last 5 years, significant emphasis has been placed on maternal quality outcomes and costs of care. Improving the quality of maternity care could dramatically reduce health care costs.[1] Despite the lack of transparency, quality metrics for maternity care are not widely adopted and reported. There has also been increased media coverage focused on the quality of maternity care and increasing maternal morbidity and mortality, including, but not limited to, *The New York Times*, *USA Today*, and *National Public Radio*.[2–5] This review discusses current

Disclosure Statement: The author has nothing to disclose.
Graduate Program, Louisiana State University Health School of Nursing, New Orleans, LA, USA
* 224 W. Greens Drive, Baton Rouge, LA, 70810.
E-mail address: mmahe4@lsuhsc.edu

challenges of increasing maternal morbidity and mortality, reporting quality metrics, rising costs, and the impetus for standardizing and regionalizing maternity care, including integrated behavioral health and preconception care.

BACKGROUND

Over the last 5 years, significant emphasis has been placed on the quality outcomes and costs of obstetric care when compared with other developed countries. The Centers for Disease Control and Prevention (CDC) Pregnancy Mortality Surveillance System reported that between 2000 and 2013, pregnancy-related mortality has increased by 20%.[6] According to the CDC, pregnancy-related deaths increased in the United States from 7.2 deaths per 100,000 live births in 1987 to 18.0 deaths per 100,000 live births in 2014.[6] The CDC defines pregnancy-related death as "as the death of a woman while pregnant or within 1 year of the end of a pregnancy, regardless of the outcome, duration, or site of the pregnancy, from any cause related to or aggravated by the pregnancy or its management, but not from accidental or incidental causes."[6] The CDC reports that approximately 700 women die each year as a result of complications during their pregnancy and/or delivery.[7] The leading causes of pregnancy-related deaths are cardiovascular disease (15.2%), noncardiovascular diseases (14.7%), infection (12.8%), and postpartum hemorrhage (PPH; 11.5%).[7]

In addition to the increased maternal mortalities, the incidence of severe maternal morbidity (SMM) is also increasing. According to the CDC, the rate of SMM increased approximately 200% from 1993 to 2014 from 49.5 SMM events per 10,000 delivery hospitalizations to 144.0 SMM events per 10,000 delivery hospitalizations.[8] An SMM event is defined by the CDC as unexpected maternal outcomes of labor and delivery that result in significant short- and long-term consequences to a woman's health and includes approximately 18 indicators (**Table 1**).[9] The CDC uses administrative hospital discharge data that include diagnosis and procedure codes from the *International Classification of Diseases, Tenth Revision (ICD-10)*. The most frequent indicator is blood transfusions due to hemorrhage, which increased by 399% from 1993 to 2014.[10] The rate of SMM in women with multiple chronic conditions is 4 times higher than in women without those conditions attributed to complications from chronic conditions.[11]

DEFINING QUALITY IN MATERNITY CARE

In 2009, The Joint Commission (TJC) convened a panel of experts to replace the pregnancy and related condition measure set to adopt measures endorsed by the National Quality Forum (NQF).[12] The current perinatal care measures include early elective delivery, cesarean birth, antenatal steroids, health care–associated bloodstream infections in newborns, and exclusive breast feeding.[12] In 2019, a new measure was introduced to capture unexpected complications in term newborns.[13]

In 2012, a set of maternity care quality measures was developed as a result of collaboration of the Physician Consortium for Performance Improvement targeting the goal of improving care for women during pregnancy, delivery, and postpartum.[14] This Maternity Care Work Group (MCMG) was assembled by the American Congress of Obstetricians and Gynecologists (ACOG), the National Committee for Quality Assurance, and the American Medical Association. Some of the outcome measures that were developed included (a) ending preventable morbidity, mortality, (b) reducing infections, (c) reducing unnecessary procedures that may cause harm or risk for both mother and baby, and (d) reducing depression, substance use during and after pregnancy (maternity care measurement set).[14] The process measures addressed overuse

Table 1
Severe maternal morbidity indicators and *International Classification of Diseases* codes

	SMM Indicator	Diagnosis (DX) or Procedure (PR)	*ICD-10*
1.	Acute myocardial infarction	DX	I21.01, I21.02, I21.09, I21.11, I21.19, I21.21, I21.29, I21.3, I21.4, I21.9, I21.A1, and I21.A9 I22.0, I22.1, I22.2, I22.8, I22.9
1a.	Aneurysm	DX	I71.00–I71.03, I71.1, I71.2, I71.3, I71.4, I71.5, I71.6, I71.8, I71.9, I79.0
2.	Acute renal failure	DX	N17.0, N17.1, N17.2, N17.8, N17.9, O90.4
3.	Adult respiratory distress syndrome	DX	J80, J95.1, J95.2, J95.3, J95.821, J95.822, J96.00, J96.01, J96.02
4.	Amniotic fluid embolism	DX	O88.11x,[a] O88.12 (childbirth), O88.13 (puerperium)
5.	Cardiac arrest/ventricular fibrillation	DX	I46.2, I46.8, I46.9, I49.01, I49.02[b]
5a.	Conversion of cardiac rhythm	PR	5A2204Z, 5A12012
6.	Disseminated intravascular coagulation	DX	D65, D68.8, D68.9, O72.3
7.	Eclampsia	DX	O15.00, O15.02, O15.03, O15.1, O15.2, O15.9 O14.22–HELLP syndrome (HELLP), second trimester, O14.23–HELLP syndrome (HELLP), third trimester
8.	Heart failure/arrest during surgery or procedure	DX	I97.120, I97.121, I97.130, I97.131
9.	Puerperal cerebrovascular disorders	DX	I60.0x-I60.9, I61.0x-I61.9, I62.0x, I62.1, I62.9, I63.0x-I63.9, I65.0x, I65.1, I65.2x, I65.8, I65.9, I66.0x, I66.1x, I66.2x, I66.3, I66.8, I66.9, I67.1, I67.2, I67.3, I67.4, I67.5, I67.6, I67.7, I67.8x, I67.9, I68.0, I68.8, I68.9, O22.51, O22.52, O22.53, I97.810, I97.811, I97.820, I97.821, O873
10	Pulmonary edema/acute heart failure	DX	J81.0, I50.1, I50.20, I50.21, I50.23, I50.30, I50.31, I50.33, I50.40, I50.41, I50.43, I50.9 (–) Add 5th character: 0 = unspecified; 1 = acute; 2 = chronic; 3 = acute on chronic
11.	Severe anesthesia complications	DX	O74.0, O74.1, O74.2, O74.3, O89.01,[c] O89.09 O89.1, O89.2
12.	Sepsis	DX	O85 or T80.211A or T81.4XXA, or severity: R65.20 (or septic shock, see indicator "Shock") or A40.0, A40.1, A40.3, A40.8, A40.9, A41.0, A41.1, A41.2, A41.3, A41.4, A41.50, A41.51, A41.52, A41.53, A41.59, A41.81, A41.89, A41.9, A32.7

(continued on next page)

Table 1
(continued)

	SMM Indicator	Diagnosis (DX) or Procedure (PR)	ICD-10
13.	Shock	DX	O75.1, R57.0, R57.1, R57.8, R57.9, R65.21, T78.2XXA, T88.2XXA, T88.6XXA, T81.10XA, T81.11XA, T81.19XA
14.	Sickle cell disease with crisis	DX	D57.00, D57.01, D57.02, D57.211, D57.212, D57.219, D57.411, D57.412, D57.419, D57.811, D57.812, D57.819
15.	Air and thrombotic embolism	DX	I26.01, I26.02, I26.09, I26.90, I26.92, I26.99 O88.011-O88.019, O88.02, O88.03, O88.211-O88.219, O88.22, O88.23, O88.311-O88.319, O88.32, O88.33, O88.81, O88.82, O88.83
16.	Blood transfusion	PR	99.0x → 160 ICD-10-PCS codes
17.	Hysterectomy	PR	0UT90ZZ, 0UT94ZZ, 0UT97ZZ, 0UT98ZZ, 0UT9FZZ
18.	Temporary tracheostomy	PR	0B110Z4, 0B110F4, 0B113Z4, 0B113F4, 0B114Z4, 0B114F4
18a.	Ventilation	PR	5A1935Z, 5A1945Z, 5A1955Z

[a] x = first, second, and third trimester.
[b] Ventricular flutter.
[c] Retained to keep as a code due to difficulties of separation from aspiration pneumonitis.
Adapted from Centers for Disease Control and Prevention. Severe maternal morbidity indicators and corresponding ICD codes during delivery hospitalizations. Available at: https://www.cdc.gov/reproductivehealth/maternalinfanthealth/smm/severe-morbidity-ICD.htm. Accessed December 13, 2018.

of services/treatments, patient safety, underuse of services/treatments, and underuse of patient-centered care strategies.[14] Still, there is a limited amount of data related to maternal outcomes that would provide a national framework for monitoring, improving, and reporting performance.[14]

In addition, the NQF reviewed 22 perinatal measures and ultimately endorsed 14 quality measures in 2012.[15] The endorsement asserted that the lower quality of care delivered during pregnancy, childbirth, and postpartum can result in preventable harm, wasted resources, prolonged length of stay (LOS), and costly intensive care admissions.[15] In addition to those adopted by TJC, NQF adopted measures, including incidence of episiotomy, timely cesarean section prophylaxis, deep vein thrombosis prophylaxis, newborn hepatitis vaccination, intrapartum group B streptococcus prophylaxis, delivery of infant less than 1500 g at appropriate level of care, sepsis in low-birth-weight infants, infants referred for retinopathy screening, and preconception care.[15]

However, despite the publication of numerous evidence-based quality metrics, there does not seem to be as much scrutiny or transparency by the Centers for Medicare and Medicaid Services (CMS) as compared with metrics, for example, elderly patients.[16] CMS funds nearly half of the 4 million births via Medicaid dollars.[16] The CMS Web site for consumers, Hospital Compare, has only one measure related to maternity care quality, early elective delivery, out of the 57 measures reported.[17]

COST OF MATERNITY CARE

With 6 million women becoming pregnant each year, pregnancy and newborn claims have a significant cost impact on commercial and government payers.[18] Providing preconception care can decrease costs, with estimates for every dollar spent, $1.60 can be saved in maternal and infant care costs.[18] The challenge is identifying the preconception period; women aged 15 to 44 years should be considered in this group because only approximately 51% of pregnancies are actually intended.[18] Preconception care can reduce complications of pregnancy, birth defects, and long-term developmental delays in the newborn.[18]

Opportunities related to utilization and cost of maternity care include reducing the primary cesarean delivery rate.[1] Women undergoing a primary cesarean delivery have increased morbidity, including ruptured uterus, unplanned hysterectomy, blood transfusions, and intensive care unit (ICU) admission.[19] The MCMG described the cost impact of maternal care services and procedures. Six out of the 15 most commonly performed procedures are attributed to childbirth and account for most patient charges.[14] Cesarean deliveries are the most commonly performed procedure in the United States and contribute to 45% of the total costs of charges related to childbirth.[14] In addition, when cesarean deliveries are performed as a result of an elective induction, the baby may spend time in the neonatal intensive care unit (NICU) and experience long-term sequelae, such as developmental delays.[1]

In a 2013 publication, *The Cost of Having a Baby in the United States*, prepared by Truven Analytics, an analysis was performed of payments for maternal and newborn care by commercial insurers and Medicaid.[20] The report analyzed claims data from more than 362,000 commercial insurance beneficiaries and more than 208,000 Medicaid enrollees from 2010. Some of the key findings included that total payments for cesarean births for commercial insurance ($27,866 vs $18,329) and Medicaid ($13,590 vs $9131) were 50% higher than for a vaginal birth.[20] From 2004 to 2010, commercial insurance payments increased 49% for vaginal births and 41% for cesarean births.[20]

The impact of SMM affects the cost of care for newborns. Often a medically indicated induction of labor is required, resulting in a preterm birth.[21] SMM is associated with hypertension, and the chance of a preterm birth has been reported as high as 53% in these women as compared with a 19% chance in women without SMM.[21] In 2014, the March of Dimes published a report stating that the average cost of an infant less than 37 weeks' gestation and/or less than 2500 g was $55,393 as compared with $5085 for a healthy full-term infant.[22]

The cost impact of SMM was described in a review of 2013 to 2014 data from the National Inpatient Sample specifically in pregnant women with multiple chronic conditions.[11] Findings revealed that the rate of SMM and maternal mortality in women with chronic conditions was 4 times higher than in women with no chronic conditions, resulting in significantly higher health care costs and utilization.[11] The additional mean cost of SMM in a woman with no chronic conditions was $4500, with one chronic condition was $5500, and with multiple chronic conditions was $7700.[11]

The cost impact of a PPH is driven by increases in the LOS, cost of blood products, medications and supplies, and added procedures.[23] In a retrospective analysis of the National Inpatient Sample database, deliveries occurring from 2012 to 2013 classified as a PPH were included along with deliveries not classified as such. The average LOS difference was 0.97 days (P<.001).[23] Of the maternal mortality events, 27.6% (16/58) were attributed to PPH.[23] Marshall and colleagues[23] described an oral communication by Carl Rose, MD, who asserted that as a result of increased LOS in the event of PPH there is an associated annual increase in costs of $106.7 million.

MAJOR CAUSES OF SEVERE MATERNAL MORBIDITY AND MORTALITY
Hypertensive Disorders of Pregnancy

Hypertensive disorders of pregnancy (HDP) affect maternal outcomes and are associated with a higher rate of SMM events.[24] The hypertensive disorders include preeclampsia-eclampsia, chronic hypertension (of any cause), chronic hypertension with superimposed preeclampsia, and gestational hypertension (**Box 1**).[25] HPD affects approximately 5% to 10% of all pregnancies and increases the incidence and the likelihood of early-onset significant cardiovascular disease, including heart failure, cardiovascular disease, renal failure, pulmonary edema, stroke, and venous thromboembolism.[21,26] There is an associated risk of cardiovascular disease in patients with HDP that requires routine screening after delivery by their primary care provider for 1 to 10 years.[24]

Preeclampsia is a pregnancy disorder associated with new onset of hypertension after 20 weeks' gestation most often accompanied by new-onset proteinuria.[27] Risk factors for preeclampsia include nulliparity, history of preeclampsia, diabetes chronic hypertension, prepregnancy body mass index greater than 30, kidney disease, and advanced maternal age.[27] However, most cases occur in healthy nulliparous women without risk factors.[27]

Box 1
Hypertensive disorders of pregnancy

Chronic hypertension	High blood pressure (BP) known to predate conception or that occurs before 20 wk' gestation
Chronic hypertension with superimposed preeclampsia	Superimposed preeclampsia is diagnosed when the woman experiences (a) a sudden exacerbation of hypertension, (b) the sudden onset of symptoms, such as increased liver enzymes, (c) a decrease in platelets, (d) develops right upper quadrant pain and severe headaches, (e) has pulmonary congestion or edema, (f) develops renal insufficiency, and/or (g) has sudden and substantial increases in protein excretion. There are subcategories described as with or without severe features
Gestational hypertension	New onset of BP elevations after 20 wk' gestation.
Preeclampsia	New onset of hypertension and proteinuria. In the absence of proteinuria, there may be thrombocytopenia and impaired liver function. There are subcategories described as with or without severe features
Eclampsia	The convulsive phase of the disorder and represents a severe sign of the disease process. It can occur with or without warning signs and symptoms, such as headache and/or hyperreflexia
Postpartum hypertension	Preeclampsia, preeclampsia, and eclampsia can develop in the postpartum period up to 6 mo' postpartum

Data from Task Force on Hypertension in Pregnancy. Classification of hypertensive disorders. Available at: https://www.acog.org/~/media/Task%20Force%20and%20Work%20Group%20Reports/public/HypertensioninPregnancy.pdf. Accessed December 5, 2018.

Chronic hypertension in pregnancy is present in approximately 0.9% to 1.5% of pregnant women and is the cause of maternal, fetal, and neonatal morbidity and mortality.[28] Chronic hypertension in pregnancy is defined as hypertension diagnosed or present before pregnancy or before 20 weeks' gestation.[29] The rate of chronic hypertension increased by 67% from 2000 to 2009 and was attributed to an increase in obesity and an increase in maternal age.[28(pe26)] Chronic hypertension is associated with an increased risk of diabetes and may be a result of obesity in this population.[28] There is an increased risk for a planned cesarean and increased risk for PPH.[30] Maternal risks of chronic hypertension in pregnancy include death, stroke, and myocardial infarction.[28] Fetal and neonatal risks include stillbirth, growth restriction, preterm birth, and congenital anomalies.[28]

A pregnant patient presenting with a confirmed acute episode of severe hypertension should be treated with antihypertensive medications within 30 to 60 minutes to prevent congestive heart failure, myocardial ischemia, and renal injury or failure.[27] Mode of delivery and anesthesia considerations depend on the gestational age and severity of disease progression. Although a vaginal delivery is preferred, a successful medical induction is unlikely with a fetal gestation of 32 weeks or less.[27] Evidence-based tool kits to treat preeclampsia are available to provide standardized treatments for improving care, such as the Preeclampsia Toolkit published by the California Maternal Quality Care Collaborative (CMQCC).[31] Finally, because preeclampsia may not manifest itself until the postpartum period and beyond discharge, patients must be diligently educated about the signs and symptoms to immediately report to their health care provider.[27]

Infections and Sepsis

Infections and sepsis represent some of the leading causes of maternal mortality.[6] The incidence of maternal morbidity and mortality due to sepsis is increasing in the United States.[32,33] In the United States from 2009 to 2011, the rates of pregnancy-related mortality increased because of an increase of deaths from infection and sepsis mostly attributed to the H1N1 influenza type A pandemic, which accounted for 12% of all pregnancy-related deaths in that time period.[6] Sepsis was the cause of 10% of the maternal deaths worldwide.[32] In 2016, the definition of sepsis was revised to highlight the lethal nature of sepsis as a life-threatening organ dysfunction caused by a dysregulated host response to infection.[34]

Analyzing delivery data from the Nationwide Inpatient Sample for the years of 1998 to 2008, the incidence of sepsis complicated 1:3333 deliveries; severe sepsis complicated 1:10,823 deliveries, and sepsis-related deaths complicated 1:105,263 deliveries.[32] The analysis described an association of severe sepsis with stillbirth, preterm delivery, PPH, and cesarean delivery in labor.[32] During the study period, the increase in severe sepsis was 112% and the increase in sepsis-related deaths was 129%.[32] Patients with severe sepsis experienced organ dysfunction that comprised respiratory dysfunction (34.2%), coagulation abnormalities (19.2%), cardiovascular dysfunction (11.6%), hepatic dysfunction (10.3%), and central nervous system dysfunction (8.2%).[32] Chronic comorbidities also contribute to sepsis risk and are associated with severe sepsis requiring diligence by providers to assess and treat sepsis appropriately and aggressively. Sociodemographic contributions, such as low socioeconomic status, require further study.[35]

There is still controversy using systemic inflammatory response syndrome, sepsis-related organ failure assessment, and/or quick sepsis-related organ failure assessment to recognize signs of maternal sepsis because of vital sign and laboratory findings associated with pregnancy.[36] There is a lack of an accepted definition for maternal sepsis, which has led to the delay in diagnosis and prompt treatment.[36] In a review of maternal sepsis, suboptimal or delayed intensive care was a factor in maternal deaths.[37] Caring for obstetric patients in the ICU is challenging especially for patients with viable pregnancies.[37] Consideration for the fetus in antenatal sepsis should include regular assessments, multidisciplinary team planning, and treatment with betamethasone if the infant is less than 34 weeks' gestation.[36]

Postpartum Hemorrhage

A hemorrhage in the postpartum period remains one of the leading causes of SMM and maternal mortality, and the incidence appears to be increasing.[38–40] ACOG defines maternal hemorrhage as a cumulative blood loss of $\geq$1000 mL of blood loss accompanied by signs or symptoms of hypovolemia within 24 hours of giving birth.[41] Hemorrhage risk tools, however, have been determined to have a specificity of just less than 60%.[41] Furthermore, 1% of women in the low-risk group experienced a severe PPH (ACOG 183).[41] In an analysis of data from the Nationwide Inpatient Sample from 1995 through 2005, 25,654 women were classified as having PPH, producing a PPH rate of 2.93 per 1000 deliveries.[42] Of those PPH cases, uterine atony accounted for 79% of the total cases with many of the patients not having any antepartum risk factors.[42]

Women undergoing a cesarean delivery are more likely to have a PPH than women experiencing a vaginal delivery.[42] In a secondary analysis of women with PPH after cesarean section from 2002 through 2012 at a tertiary obstetric center in the United States, 2 cohorts were developed for review: women undergoing a prelabor cesarean delivery (n = 269) versus an intrapartum cesarean delivery (n = 278).[43] In the prelabor cesarean delivery cohort, of those women with severe PPH, 18% of the women had a cesarean hysterectomy and 72% of those were the result of an abnormal implantation of the placenta and represented 49% of the ICU admissions.[43] In the intrapartum cesarean delivery cohort, 4% of the women had a hysterectomy. In the intrapartum cesarean delivery group, the ICU admission rate was 10%, and 6% of those women required mechanical ventilation for respiratory failure.[43]

In October 2017, ACOG published a revised practice bulletin outlining the guidelines for clinical management of PPH.[41] The guidelines reinforce the need for all obstetric units to use published algorithms when evaluating, treating, and monitoring patients with PPH.[41] Hospitals should adopt a systematic approach to PPH in 4 categories, including response readiness, recognition and prevention, multidisciplinary response team, and system-based quality improvement processes to review PPH events.[41]

IMPROVING MATERNAL OUTCOMES
Regionalized Maternity Care Levels

As far back as the 1970s, studies revealed that the appropriate and timely delivery of risk-based obstetric and neonatal care resulted in improved maternal outcomes.[44] In 1976, the March of Dimes published, "Toward Improving the Outcomes of Pregnancy," that defined levels of maternal and neonatal care and provided guidance regarding the necessary resources and personnel to address the complexity of care required to deliver safe and effective care.[44] Since this publication, most of the focus on regionalization of health care services defined in Guidelines for Perinatal Care has been on neonatal care.[44] However, with the increase in maternal mortality over the last 14 years, more emphasis on maternal levels of care is required so that maternal transfers can be prioritized to provide the appropriate level of care for high-risk mothers.[44] The evidence suggests that obstetric complications are more prevalent in hospitals with lower delivery volumes.[44]

In 2015, ACOG and the Society for Maternal Fetal Medicine published "Levels of Maternal Care" to provide (a) definitions for levels of maternity care, (b) guidelines for quality and health promotion for maternity care levels, and (c) development of equitable distribution of full service maternity care services.[44] In addition, the document provided clarification on the types of capabilities and types of health care providers required for each level of maternity care in birth centers, level 1, level 2, level 3, and level 4 centers.[44] There is limited research on the outcomes of the standardization of regionalization of maternity care, so monitoring SMM and mortality events becomes even more critical. Finally, it will possibly require state and/or national accrediting bodies to establish, monitor, and finance these centers.[44] In a review of 9 maternal morbidity review committees, evidence supports adopting levels of maternal care as described by ACOG and Society for Maternal-Fetal Medicine so that the appropriate effective and timely care for complications of maternal care can be delivered.[45]

Maternal Quality Collaborative Tool Kits and Safety Bundles

In 2011, the CMQCC and the state of California published its first critical analysis of pregnancy-related deaths that occurred from 2002 through 2007.[46] As a result of this analysis, quality improvement opportunities were identified and provided the stimulus for the development of evidence-based quality improvement tool kits.[46] The tool kits include cardiovascular disease, preeclampsia, early elective delivery, hemorrhage, maternal venous thromboembolism, and supporting vaginal birth and reducing primary cesarean deliveries.[46]

As previously described, obstetric hemorrhage has increased most significantly as compared with other SMM events and remains one of the leading causes of maternal death.[47] The CMQCC first published the tool kit in 2010 and was revised in 2015. California hospitals that participated in hemorrhage collaboratives realized a 20.8% reduction in maternal morbidity related to hemorrhage as compared with 1.2% reduction in nonparticipating hospitals.[48] Nevertheless, the data regarding the implementation of hemorrhage tool kits across the United States in hospitals that provide maternity care are not known.

The Council on Patient Safety in Women's Health Care (CPSWHC) is a national partnership of organizations that has defined its purpose to reduce harm by supporting investigation of harm, implementing patient safety initiatives, providing education, and supporting transparency and accountability.[49] The council has developed maternal safety bundles for maternal mental health, venous thromboembolism, opioid use disorders, hemorrhage, postpartum care basics, prevention of retained vaginal sponges, reducing disparities, reducing primary cesarean birth, severe hypertension, maternal morbidity reviews, and support after severe maternal events. The patient safety bundles consist of a framework defining readiness for every unit, recognition and prevention for every patient, response for every event, and reporting and systems learning on every unit.

The CPSWHC is positioned to achieve its purpose with the development of the Alliance for Innovation on Maternal Health (AIM).[50] AIM is a national data-driven maternal safety and quality improvement initiative with a goal to eliminate preventable SMM and maternal mortality.[50] States willing to participate must have a maternal mortality review committee that is willing to submit data. Although states can initiate multiple maternal safety bundles, it is recommended to implement only 1 bundle at a time until implementation and monitoring are established.

In 2017, the CDC and March of Dimes launched the National Network of Perinatal Quality Collaboratives to support state-based Perinatal Quality Collaboratives (PQCs).[51] Improvements achieved by state or multistate PQC include reductions in early elective deliveries, health care–associated bloodstream infections in newborns, and severe pregnancy complications. In addition, the CDC is providing additional financial support to reduce preterm births, severe pregnancy complications, racial/ethnic disparities, and cesarean births in the states of Colorado, Delaware, Florida, Georgia, Illinois, Louisiana, Massachusetts, Minnesota, Mississippi, New Jersey, New York, Oregon, and Wisconsin.[51]

Simulation

An essential part of the safety bundles and tool kits is the use of simulation to improve outcomes of pregnancy-related complications.[52] The 3 areas of simulation focus include skill acquisition, interval training, and in situ drills.[52] A reduction in blood transfusions was demonstrated after implementation of PPH simulation drills in obstetric units.[53,54] Between 2005 and 2008, 3 small community hospitals participated in a study with 1 hospital serving as the control group and 2 hospitals serving as intervention sites.[55] One intervention site hospital participated in the TeamSTEPPS program, and the second intervention site hospital had both TeamSTEPPS didactic training and unit-based simulation training.[55] A statistically significant decrease in perinatal morbidity (37%) was realized at the hospital site that performed routine simulation along with TeamSTEPPS training.[55]

Maternal Early Warning Criteria

With 40% to 50% of maternal deaths deemed potentially preventable, an effective early warning system to timely recognize signs of deterioration in women with complications is crucial. For the last 2 decades, several tools have been developed to track observations and define criteria to trigger the identification of pending complications, including the Obstetric Early Warning Score, Modified Early Obstetric Warning System (MEOWS), and the Maternal Early Warning Criteria (MEWC).[56–58] Multiple studies to validate the tools have been conducted and require further research. Nevertheless, the universal adoption of hospitals providing obstetric care has not been established.[56–58]

In 2014, the National Partnership for Maternal Safety published a proposal to adopt the MEWC as an efficient way to timely identify maternal morbidity to prevent mortality.[59] Previously developed tools require significant time and burden or lack specificity to be clinically useful.[59] For example, the MEOWS included normal, amber or caution, and red or urgent parameters. Adapted from the red triggers in the MEOWS, the MEWC includes measurement of systolic and diastolic blood pressure, heart rate, respiratory rate, oxygen saturation, oliguria, maternal agitation, confusion or unresponsiveness, and reported headache or shortness of breath in a patient with preeclampsia.[59] More research is required, which could be facilitated by the adoption of such tools.

Severe Maternal Morbidity and Mortality Reviews

In December 2018, a bill, Preventing Maternal Mortality Act, was passed by the US House and US Senate and was signed into law by the President authorizing more than $60 million over 5 years to provide funding for maternal mortality review committees in all 50 states.[60] These committees will collect data on the causes of death in women during or after childbirth. These reviews and data will include maternal deaths from suicide and homicide. Conducting reviews at the organization and state level will elucidate opportunities for improvement.

Conducting reviews of SMM and maternal mortality at the organizational level are required by TJC. Hospitals should have multidisciplinary standing committees with representation of obstetric care providers, anesthesia, nursing, quality improvement specialists, administration, and patient advocates. Timely and systematic reviews should be conducted to ascertain system, provider, and patient factors that contributed to the event.[61] System and provider factors to be reviewed include the point of access to care, diagnosis, referral, treatment, team communication, policies and procedures, documentation, equipment and environmental factors, and discharge. Patient factors include a review of prepregnancy conditions, previous obstetric conditions, nonobstetric medical complications, behavioral health, significant stressors, and barriers to access of health care.

Conducting reviews of SMM and maternal mortality at the state level is critical in the prevention of maternal mortality.[62] The Association of Maternal and Child Health Programs developed the resource, Review to Action, that provides a framework to support state maternal mortality reviews. The CDC Division of Reproductive Health and the CDC Foundation's Review to Action are the result of a larger initiative, "Building US Capacity to Review and Prevent Maternal Deaths," and include the Maternal Mortality Review Information Application (MMRIA). MMRIA supports the standardization of data abstraction, case narrative development, committee decisions, and analysis.[62] According to MMRIA, only half of the states in the United States have a state-sponsored maternal mortality review committee.[62] A framework for conducting mortality reviews was developed to guide data abstraction processes and facilitate probing questions to determine system process improvement.[63]

Pregnancy Care Management

The implementation of care management programs has the potential to improve maternal quality outcomes related to improving overall prenatal care and lowering preterm birth rates and postpartum care.[64] In 2012, the Community Care of North Carolina program published a pregnancy care management standardized plan (PCMSP).[65] The document defines pregnancy care management as a "collaborative set of interventions and activities, including assessment, planning, facilitation, care coordination, evaluation and advocacy for options and services that address the healthcare and preventive service needs of pregnant and postpartum women through communication and available resources to promote quality, cost effective outcomes."[65(p1)]

The North Carolina PCMSP identified priority risk criteria to identify the target population for care management services and referrals, including, but not limited to, multiple gestation, fetal complications, maternal chronic conditions, substance misuse, history of preterm birth or low birth rate, late prenatal care, and unsafe living conditions.[65] The pathways during the prenatal period include access, referrals and education, provider collaboration, and monitoring.[65] During the postpartum period, pathways include access, referrals and education, and provider collaboration.[65]

Behavioral Health Integration

In the United States, clinical depression is the leading cause of disability in women of reproductive age.[66] Perinatal depression is defined as either minor or major depression occurring during pregnancy and/or up to 12 months after delivery.[67] The incidence of postpartum depression is more likely in women who experience medical complications and/or a premature delivery.[68] It is estimated that 5% to more than 25% of new mothers experience postpartum depression.[69]

A measure of maternity care quality includes conducting a behavioral health risk assessment in the prenatal period.[14] The risk assessment should occur during the first prenatal visit using a validated tool. The assessment should include screening for depression, alcohol use, tobacco use, illicit drug use, and intimate partner violence.[14] This screening is recommended to be conducted at prescribed intervals because women may not admit to any issues the first time that they are asked, and their individual situation may change.

Positive behavioral health screening results require interventions, such as behavioral counseling, tobacco cessation resources, mandatory reporting requirements, and referrals to agencies. The compelling need to perform screening for illicit drug use cannot be stressed enough considering that women with a history of substance misuse have an increased suicide risk by 11 times[70] or 2.5 to 2.6 deaths per 100,000 births.[71] Equally compelling is the need for screening for intimate partner violence due to risk of pregnancy-associated homicide risk ranging from 2.2 to 6.2 deaths per 100,000 births.[42]

Behavioral health care integration in primary care is gaining traction, providing mental health and substance use services.[72] With the stigmatization associated with seeking mental health services, many women forgo seeking treatment. Therefore, integrating behavioral health care resources in obstetric and gynecologic care settings will provide a framework for a team approach to meet the mother's medical and behavioral health needs.

SUMMARY

The quality of maternal care delivered must be made a priority at the local, regional, state, and national level. The increasing incidence of maternal morbidity and mortality requires the implementation of evidence-based practices. Maternal mortality review committees at the organizational and state levels must have nursing representation to identify system process failures and implement system level process improvements. Nurses providing care to this patient population must be competent, participate in simulation, and advocate for the adoption of evidence-based care. Nurses have the obligation to be active politically especially when it comes to funding resources to provide access to health care for women of childbearing age. For those nurses working in organizations providing the highest levels of maternity care, it is imperative to provide educational outreach to nurses in centers providing lower levels of care. Finally, there must be more accountability and transparency regarding the utilization of evidence-based care, costs, and the outcomes of maternal care.

REFERENCES

1. Maternity care. Center for Healthcare Quality & Payment Reform website. Available at: http://www.chqpr.org/maternitycare.html. Accessed December 18, 2018.
2. Tavernise S. Maternal mortality rate in U.S. rises, defying global trend, study finds. 2016. Available at: https://www.nytimes.com/2016/09/22/health/maternal-mortality.html?_r=0. Accessed December 5, 2018.
3. National Public Radio. Nearly dying in childbirth: why preventable complications are growing in U.S. 2017. Available at: https://www.npr.org/2017/12/22/572298802/nearly-dying-in-childbirth-why-preventable-complications-are-growing-in-u-s. Accessed December 5, 2018.
4. National Public Radio. For every woman who dies in childbirth in the U.S., 70 more come close. 2018. Available at: https://www.npr.org/2018/05/10/607782992/for-every-woman-who-dies-in-childbirth-in-the-u-s-70-more-come-close. Accessed December 5, 2018.

5. Chuck E. NBC News. She died after birth. Her grieving husband hopes a new bill will save others 2018. Available at: https://www.msn.com/en-us/health/medical/she-died-after-giving-birth-her-grieving-husband-hopes-a-new-bill-will-save-others/ar-BBRavxi?li=BBnb7Kz. Accessed December 20, 2018.
6. Pregnancy mortality surveillance system. 2018. Centers for Disease Control and Prevention website. Available at: https://www.cdc.gov/reproductivehealth/maternalinfanthealth/pregnancy-mortality-surveillance-system.htm. Accessed December 5, 2018.
7. Pregnancy-related deaths. 2018. Centers for Disease Control and Prevention website. Available at: https://www.cdc.gov/reproductivehealth/maternalinfanthealth/pregnancy-relatedmortality.htm. Accessed December 5, 2018.
8. Severe maternal morbidity in the United States. 2017. Centers for Disease Control and Prevention website. Available at: https://www.cdc.gov/reproductivehealth/maternalinfanthealth/severematernalmorbidity.html. Accessed December 7, 2018.
9. Severe maternal morbidity indicators and corresponding ICD codes during delivery hospitalizations. 2018. Centers for Disease Control and Prevention website. Available at: https://www.cdc.gov/reproductivehealth/maternalinfanthealth/smm/severe-morbidity-ICD.htm. Accessed December 5, 2018.
10. Rates in severe morbidity indicators per 10,000 delivery hospitalizations. 2018. Centers for Disease Control and Prevention website. Available at: https://www.cdc.gov/reproductivehealth/maternalinfanthealth/smm/severe-morbidity-ICD.htm. Accessed December 7, 2018.
11. Admon LK, Winkelman TN, Heisler M, et al. Obstetric outcomes and delivery-related health care utilization and costs among pregnant women with multiple chronic conditions. 2018. Centers for Disease Control and Prevention website. Available at: https://www.cdc.gov/pcd/issues/2018/17_0397.htm. Accessed December 31, 2018.
12. Specifications manual for Joint Commission quality measures: perinatal care. The Joint Commission website. Available at: https://manual.jointcommission.org/releases/TJC2018A1/PerinatalCare.html. Accessed December 17, 2018.
13. Specifications manual for Joint Commission quality measures: perinatal care. The Joint Commission website. Available at: https://manual.jointcommission.org/releases/TJC2018B1/PerinatalCare.html. Accessed December 17, 2018.
14. Maternity care performance measurement set. American Congress of Obstetricians and Gynecologists, National Committee for Quality Assurance, and Physician Consortium for Performance Improvement®. 2012. Agency for Healthcare Reform and Quality website. Available at: https://www.ahrq.gov/sites/default/files/wysiwyg/CHIPRA-BMI-Maternity-Care-Measures.pdf. Accessed December 12, 2018.
15. NQF endorses perinatal measures. 2012. National quality forum website. Available at: http://www.qualityforum.org/news_and_resources/press_releases/2012/nqf_endorses_perinatal_measures.aspx. Accessed December 17, 2018.
16. Young A. USA Today. Hospitals know how to protect mothers. They just aren't doing it. 2018. Available at: https://www.usatoday.com/in-depth/news/investigations/deadly-deliveries/2018/07/26/maternal-mortality-rates-preeclampsia-postpartum-hemorrhage-safety/546889002/. Accessed December 31, 2018.
17. Measures and current data collection periods. 2018. Medicare.gov: hospital compare website. Available at: https://www.medicare.gov/hospitalcompare/Data/Data-Updated.html#. Accessed December 31, 2018.

18. Maternal and child health: a business imperative. Business Group on Health website. Available at: https://www.businessgrouphealth.org/pub/?id=f2ffff14-2354-d714-51f4-86f969e42856. Accessed January 1, 2019.

19. Maternal morbidity for vaginal and cesarean deliveries, according to previous cesarean history: new data from the Birth Certificate, 2013. Natl Vital Stat Rep 2015; 64(4):1–13. Available at: https://www.cdc.gov/nchs/data/nvsr/nvsr64/nvsr64_04.pdf. Accessed December 17, 2018.

20. The cost of having a baby in the United States. Truven health analytics. 2013. Childbirth Connection website. Available at: http://transform.childbirthconnection.org/wp-content/uploads/2013/01/Cost-of-Having-a-Baby1.pdf. Accessed December 31, 2018.

21. Hitti J, Sienas L, Walker S, et al. Contribution of hypertension to severe maternal morbidity. Am J Obstet Gynecol 2018;219:405.e1-7. Available at: https://doi.org/10.1016/j.ajog.2018.07.002. Accessed December 19, 2018.

22. Premature babies cost employers $12.7 billion annually. 2014. March of Dimes website. Available at: https://www.marchofdimes.org/news/premature-babies-cost-employers-127-billion-annually.aspx. Accessed December 31, 2018.

23. Marshall AL, Durani U, Bartley A, et al. The impact of postpartum hemorrhage on hospital length of stay and inpatient mortality: a National Inpatient Sample-based analysis. Am J Obstet Gynecol 2017;217:344.e1-6.

24. Ying W, Catov JM, Ouyang P. Hypertensive disorders of pregnancy and future maternal cardiovascular risk. J Am Heart Assoc 2018;7:1–9.

25. Task Force on hypertension in pregnancy. Classification of hypertensive disorders. 2013. American College of Obstetricians and Gynecologists website. Available at: https://www.acog.org/~/media/Task%20Force%20and%20Work%20Group%20Reports/public/HypertensioninPregnancy.pdf. Accessed December 5, 2018.

26. Stevens W, Shih T, Incerti D, et al. Short term costs of preeclampsia to the United States health care system. Am J Obstet Gynecol 2017;4(32):237–48.

27. ACOG practice bulletin No. 202: gestational hypertension and preeclampsia. Obstet Gynecol 2019;133:e1–25.

28. ACOG practice bulletin No. 203: chronic hypertension in pregnancy. Obstet Gynecol 2019;133:e26–50.

29. Bateman BT, Bansil P, Hernandez-Diaz S, et al. Prevalence, trends, and outcomes of chronic hypertension: a nationwide sample of delivery admissions. Am J Obstet Gynecol 2012;206(2):134.e1-8.

30. Panaitescu AM, Syngelaki A, Prodan N, et al. Chronic hypertension and adverse pregnancy outcome: a cohort study. Ultrasound Obstet Gynecol 2011;50:228–35.

31. Improving health care response to preeclampsia: a California quality improvement toolkit. 2013. California Maternal Quality Care Collaborative website. Available at: https://www.cmqcc.org/resources-tool-kits/toolkits/. Accessed January 1, 2019.

32. Bauer ME, Bateman BT, Bauer ST, et al. Maternal sepsis mortality and morbidity during hospitalization for delivery: temporal trends and independent associations for severe sepsis. Anesth Analg 2013;117(4):944–50.

33. Maternal collapse in pregnancy and the puerperium, RCOG Green top guideline No. 56. 2011. Royal College of Obstetricians and Gynaecologists website. Available at: https://www.rcog.org.uk/globalassets/documents/guidelines/gtg_56.pdf. Accessed January 2, 2019.

34. Singer M, Deutschman CS, Seymour CW, et al. The third international consensus definitions for sepsis and septic shock (sepsis-3). J Am Med Assoc 2016;315(8):801–10.

35. Acosta CD, Harrison DA, Rowan K, et al. Maternal morbidity and mortality from severe sepsis. A national cohort study. BMJ Open 2016;6:e012323.
36. Vaught AJ. Maternal sepsis. Semin Perinatol 2018;42:9–12.
37. Hashmi M, Khan FH. A review of critical care management of maternal sepsis. Anaesth Pain Intensive Care 2014;18(4):430–5.
38. Merriam AA, Wright JD, Siddiq Z, et al. Risk for postpartum hemorrhage, transfusion, and hemorrhage related morbidity at low, moderate and high volume hospitals. J Matern Fetal Neonatal Med 2017;31(8):1025–34.
39. Miller CM, Cohn S, Akdagli S, et al. Postpartum hemorrhage following vaginal delivery: risk factors and maternal outcomes. J Perinatol 2017;37:243–8.
40. Main EK, Cape V, Abreo A, et al. Reduction of severe maternal morbidity from hemorrhage using a state perinatal quality collaborative. Am J Obstet Gynecol 2017;216:298e1–11.
41. Committee on Practice Bulletins-Obstetrics. Practice bulletin No. 183: postpartum hemorrhage. Obstet Gynecol 2017;130:e168-86.
42. Bateman BT, Berman MF, Riley LE, et al. The epidemiology of postpartum hemorrhage in a large nationwide sample of deliveries. Int Anesth Res Soc 2010; 110(5):1368–73.
43. Seligman B, Ramachandran B, Hegde P, et al. Obstetric interventions and maternal morbidity among women who experience severe postpartum hemorrhage during cesarean delivery. Int J Obstet Anesth 2017;31:27–36.
44. Obstetric care consensus No. 2: levels of maternal care. Obstet Gynecol 2015; 125:502–15.
45. Simpson KR. Severe maternal morbidity and maternal mortality: what can be learned from reviewing near miss and adverse events? MCN Am J Matern Child Nurs 2018;43(4):240.
46. California Maternal Quality Care Collaborative: What we do. California maternal quality care collaborative website. Available at: https://www.cmqcc.org/about-cmqcc/what-we-do. Accessed December 28, 2018.
47. OB hemorrhage toolkit V 2.0: executive summary. 2015. California maternal quality care collaborative website. Available at: https://www.cmqcc.org/resources-tool-kits/toolkits/ob-hemorrhage-toolkit. Accessed December 28, 2018.
48. Hemorrhage collaboratives. California maternal quality care collaborative website. Available at: https://www.cmqcc.org/qi-initiatives/obstetric-hemorrhage/hemorrhage-collaboratives. Accessed December 31, 2018.
49. Purpose statement. Council on patient safety in Women's healthcare website. Available at: https://safehealthcareforeverywoman.org/about-us/. Accessed December 28, 2018.
50. What is AIM? Alliance for innovation on maternal health website. 2018. Available at: https://safehealthcareforeverywoman.org/aim-program/. Accessed December 31, 2018.
51. About perinatal care collaboratives. 2018. Centers for Disease Control and Prevention website. Available at: https://www.cdc.gov/reproductivehealth/maternalinfanthealth/pqc.htm. Accessed December 31, 2018.
52. Deering S. Using simulation to reduce maternal morbidity. 2018. Contemporary OB/GYN website. Available at: http://www.contemporaryobgyn.net/surgery/using-simulation-technology-improve-maternal-morbidity. Accessed January 1, 2019.
53. Rizvi F, Mackey R, Barrett T, et al. Successful reduction of massive postpartum haemorrhage by use of guidelines and staff education. Br J Obstet Gynaecol 2004;111:495–8.

54. Egenberg S, Oian P, Bru LE, et al. Can inter-professional simulation training influence the frequency of blood transfusions after birth? Acta Obstet Gynecol Scand 2015;94:316–23.

55. Riley W, Davis S, Miller K, et al. Didactic and simulation nontechnical skills team training to improve perinatal patient outcomes in a community hospital. Jt Comm J Qual Patient Saf 2011;37(8):357–8.

56. Ryan HM, Jones MA, Payne BA, et al. Validating the performance of the Modified Early Obstetric Warning System multivariable model to predict maternal intensive care unit admission. J Obstet Gynaecol Can 2017;39(9):728–33.

57. Carle C, Alexander P, Columb M, et al. Design and internal validation of an obstetric early warning score: secondary analysis of the Intensive Care National Audit and Research Centre case mix programme database. Anaesthesia 2013; 68(4):354–67.

58. Paternina-Caicedo A, Mranda J, Bourjelly G, et al. Performance of the Obstetric Early Warning Score in critically ill patients for the prediction of maternal death. AM J Obstet Gynecol 2017;216:58.e1-8.

59. Mhyre JM, D'Oria R, Hameed AB, et al. The maternal early warning criteria: a proposal from the National Partnership for Maternal Safety. J Obstet Gynecol Neonatal Nurs 2014;43:771–9.

60. Slabodkin G. Trump signs into law maternal mortality prevention legislation. 2018. Health Data Management. Available at: https://www.healthdatamanagement. com/news/trump-signs-into-law-maternal-mortality-prevention-legislation. Accessed January 1, 2019.

61. Council on patient safety in Women's health care. SMM review form v6-28-2016_long. Available at: https://safehealthcareforeverywoman.org/patient-safety-tools/severe-maternal-morbidity-review/. Accessed January 1, 2019.

62. Review to action: about us. Review to Action website. Available at: http:// reviewtoaction.org/about-us. Accessed January 1, 2019.

63. Maternal mortality review committee abstractor manual. Review to Action website. Available at: http://reviewtoaction.org/resource-search-center. Accessed January 2, 2019.

64. Bell J. Perinatal case management. Obstetric poster presentation. J Obstet Gynecol Neonatal Nurs 2016;45:S5–36.

65. Pregnancy care management standardized plan. 2012. North Carolina Public Health. Available at: https://whb.ncpublichealth.com/provPart/docs/ pregCareManual/PregnancyCareManagementStandardizedPlan-Revised2012-11-13.pdf. Accessed December 26, 2018.

66. Data on behavioral health in the United States. American Psychological Association website. Available at: https://www.apa.org/helpcenter/data-behavioral-health.aspx. Accessed December 19, 2018.

67. Depression basics. 2016. National Institute of Mental Health website. Available at: https://www.nimh.nih.gov/health/publications/depression/index.shtml. Accessed December 19, 2018.

68. Postpartum depression facts. National Institute of Mental Health website. Available at: https://www.nimh.nih.gov/health/publications/postpartum-depression-facts/index.shtml. Accessed December 19, 2018.

69. Gaynes BN, Gavin N, Meltzer-Brody S, et al. Perinatal depression: prevalence, screening accuracy, and screening outcomes: summary. In: AHRQ evidence report summaries, 119. Rockville (MD): Agency for Healthcare Research and Quality (US); 2005. p. 1998–2005. Available at: https://www.ncbi.nlm.nih.gov/ books/NBK11838/. Accessed December 19, 2018.

70. Comtois KA, Schiff MA, Grossman DC. Psychiatric risk factors associated with postpartum suicide attempt in Washington state, 1992-2001. Am J Obstet Gynecol 2008;199(2):120.e1-5.
71. Wallace ME, Hoyert D, Williams C, et al. Pregnancy related homicide and suicide in 37 US states with enhanced pregnancy surveillance. Am J Obstet Gynecol 2016;215:364.e1-10.
72. Behavioral health and primary care. 2018. Health Resources and Services Administration website. Available at: https://bphc.hrsa.gov/qualityimprovement/clinicalquality/behavioralhealth/index.html. Accessed December 19, 2018.

Pediatric Quality Metrics Related to Quality and Cost

Catherine Haut, DNP, CPNP, CCRN*, Aaron Carpenter, DNP, Mdiv, CPNP,
Jane Mericle, MHS-CL, BSN, RN, CENP

KEYWORDS

- Pediatric quality • Pediatric indicators • Pediatric measures
- Children's health quality

KEY POINTS

- Quality metrics in health care have been in use for many years; however, pediatric measures are not as well supported as those designed for adults.
- The history of measuring pediatric inpatient and outpatient health care quality continues to evolve into a unique process, with candidate measures created by multiple organizations and governmental agencies, including the Centers for Medicaid & Medicare Services.
- To pursue high-level, quality care, children's hospitals, providers, and practices are charged with developing improvement processes that evaluate current practice and offer solutions for change.
- A large children's hospital system is eager to exceed pediatric national quality indicators with the mission of providing the highest quality care and experiences for patients and their families, with the emphasis on quality and cost-saving practices.

INTRODUCTION

Major transformation in health care began more than 20 years ago with movement from payment for specific health and disease services to a focus on quality with cost containment. Financial benefit or saving is easily understood; however, quality as it relates to health care services is more difficult to comprehend, especially in the pediatric population in which errors even in simple calculations can result in serious adverse events. The term quality is defined as a standard, measure of excellence, feature, trait, or attribute that sets aside or specifies an overall or detailed expectation.[1] Quality equals reliability, an extremely important concept for health care outcomes. The National Academy of Medicine (NAM) recognize health care quality as care linked to population outcomes.[2,3] The NAM defines quality of care as "the degree

Disclosure Statement: The authors have nothing to disclose.
Nemours Alfred I Dupont Hospital for Children, 1600 Rockland Road, Wilmington, DE 19803, USA
* Corresponding author.
E-mail address: Catherine.haut@nemours.org

to which health care services for individuals and populations increase the likelihood of desired health outcomes and are consistent with current professional knowledge."[4] In 2001, the NAM identified 6 domains of quality, which include safety, effectiveness, patient-centered, timely, efficient, and equitable, and listed 10 rules for redesign of health care, incorporating a patient-focused and financially focused agenda.[3] These requirements can be applied to any arena of care, including pediatrics, and are measured based on patient population outcomes.[5]

Quality Metrics

Currently, in the health care literature, quality is described in metrics, indicators, measures, and improvement modalities. Quality metrics are specific or performance measures that have been developed to support institutional or organizational assessment, and quality improvement at the provider, hospital, or entire health care system levels.[6] Metrics are valuable provider tools, derived from evidence, including governmental or organizational data, and are used as the basis for measurements that enhance quality of care.

Quality Measures

Quality measures are important in the determination of health care outcomes. In 1966, Avedis Donabedian, a physician theorist, published a framework that categorizes quality measures as structure, process, and outcomes.[7] Donabedian processes have been endorsed by the National Quality Forum (NQF) and the Centers for Medicare and Medicaid Services (CMS).[8,9] The CMS, from which adult quality measures originated, provides the basis for pay-for-performance models, and defines quality measures as tools that measure health care processes, outcomes, and organizational structures and/or systems of care.[9] In August, 2018, the CMS published 2 new programs for children: a model to address the opioid crisis and effects on children and the Integrated Care for Kids model.[10] The latter model is focused entirely on children's health with an emphasis on early identification and treatment, integrated care coordination, and payment for performance.[10] Currently, there are candidate quality measures or metrics in pediatrics, meaning they are proposed based on evidence, such as clinical practice guidelines, but still require investigation.[11] In the CMS system, candidate measures are created through internal and external panels, offered for public comment, and finalized with consensus endorsement.[11]

The American Academy of Pediatrics (AAP) published a statement on quality in 2008 that aligns with the Agency for Healthcare Research and Quality (AHRQ), indicating that the purpose of quality measurement is to improve patient care and outcomes, including health status and satisfaction.[12] The AAP measures compare performance within the organization itself over time, with other organizations, and with exemplary institutions.[12,13] The NQF is a private sector organization referenced by the CMS that sets standards in health care quality by evaluation and endorsement of set performance measures.[14] Other arenas for measuring quality are through individual specialty organizations with pediatric-specific measures published daily as candidate measures.

Quality Indicators

Quality indicators can evaluate a process of care; provide a quantitative monitor for organizational, clinical, financial, or management functions; or represent specific tools to evaluate or improve patient outcomes.[15] As measures, indicators can have different foci and are used as guides for comparison within populations and organizations. Different types of indicators include those that are rate-based, with the example of hospital-acquired infections, or structure or process-based, which include access to specialties in care or coordination of care for illness management, such as specialty planning for children with multisystem health problems.[16]

Quality as described through structure, process, and outcome is documented on the AHRQ Web site.[16] Structural measures include systems in place to provide care, such as board-certified specialists or the ratio of providers to patients. Process measures review the number of patients who experience a specific procedure or preventative service in an organization. Outcome measures identify the impact of the health care product or service, such as how many patients died as a result of a surgical procedure and rates of hospitalization-related complications.[7,17] The American Nurses Association established indicators in 1998 more specific to nursing care quality and processes but also in line with the Donabedian framework.[18] The National Database of Nursing Quality Indicators provides hospitals with unit-level performance measured against national data; however, similar to other data, these are generic to nursing and not specific to pediatrics.[18] Quality indicators are developed based on evidence, user experience, and empirical analysis, and are reviewed by clinical panels to set definitions and measure rates.[19] Indicators in pediatrics are still new and few statistical metrics are in place.

Purpose

This article attempts to review the evolution of pediatric quality metrics and measures, and investigates pediatric quality within a large pediatric hospital. The information presented offers knowledge applicable to pediatric quality, with a history of the development of quality metrics and the evolution of specific pediatric measures. Examples of pediatric quality projects completed by a large children's hospital system are included. These projects include quality and financial initiatives that lead to improved, efficient, and sustainable patient, family, or staff outcomes.

HISTORY OF PEDIATRIC QUALITY

Quality in pediatrics or in health care in general cannot be discussed independently without first introducing the concept of evidence. Evidence-based practice (EBP) was theoretically implied in nursing by Florence Nightingale in the mid-1800s. She was credited with using evidence or observed outcomes as the basis for treatment decisions. In the 1800s, medical doctors (MDs) also used EBP until the early 1900s when trends moved to independent decision-making for treatment.[20] However, in the 1920s, when medicine began to more specifically define EBP, especially in the era of inconsistent practice between MDs, EBP became more meaningful in health care.[21] The evidence process was formalized initially in the 1960s when the Canadian physician, epidemiologist, and researcher, Dr David Sackett,[17] described EBP as the combination of research evidence with clinical skills and included the patient in management decision-making.[21] Sackett and colleagues[21] defined EBP as "the conscientious, explicit and judicious use of current best evidence in making decisions about the care of the individual patient. It means integrating individual clinical expertise with the best available external clinical evidence from systematic research." In 2000, Sackett and colleagues[21] described another concept in care, termed patient preference. EBP includes clinician expertise, best research, and patient or family preference. Pediatric research, however, has a paucity of randomized controlled trials and large-volume studies owing to the ethical issues involved with conducting experimental research with children, so using EBP in caring for children remains a challenge.

EBP in nursing reflects the same characteristics as in medicine, with current interest in including a multidisciplinary or interprofessional approach. Nursing EBP began with Florence Nightingale who examined the relationship of cleanliness and patient demographics to patient outcome.[20] According to Melnyk and colleagues[22] (2014), "EBP is an ongoing, life-long problem solving process designed to merge science and art, that integrates the best evidence, incorporating critical appraisal and synthesis of research from well-designed studies, internal evidence from QI and clinical expertise with integration of patient preferences and values." Melnyk and colleagues[22] developed and validated EBP competencies that can be used to insure quality care and outcomes within all nursing areas and patient populations.

Quality and Safety Education for Nurses

Quality and Safety Education for Nurses competencies were introduced in 2005, and updated in 2012, to be incorporated into nursing curriculum for both undergraduate and graduate-level nurses.[23] Patient-centered care, teamwork and collaboration, EBP, quality improvement, safety, and informatics are the competencies presented with the intent for nurses to have the knowledge, skills, and attitudes necessary for the quality and safety of health care systems.[23] Nurses and advanced practice nurses (APNs) are reeducated to integrate EBP and QI in practice.

The American Association of Critical Care Nurses (AACN) synergy model was developed in 1996 and forms the basis for certification examinations but is also a model that aligns patient needs with nurse competencies, which is easily applied to neonatal and pediatric populations.[24] Complexity of care is addressed from an outcomes perspective. Nursing competencies, such as critical thinking, advocacy, and caring practices, are included in the model. It also involves interdisciplinary collaboration, which is key to managing patients, especially those at risk for complications.[25] In the AACN model, clinical experience along with patient involvement creates an evidence-based process for quality.[24]

Institute of Medicine

Considering the use of evidence in nursing practice, education, and care models indicates a distinct relationship between EBP and quality of care because 1 is the basis for the other. Quality outcomes are rooted in the best evidence and quality indicators reference evidence and up-to-date research activities. The bridge between EBP and quality connects within health care quality history beginning in the 1980s with primary interests focused on containing health care costs. In 2009, the NAM was commissioned by Congress to study actual health care quality aside from financial implications and published the report, "To Err is Human: Building a Safer Health System."[26] This report highlights the concerning statistics of medical error and recommends open discussion of mistakes made by health care professionals, taking the legal or liability concerns away and replacing these with learning through evaluation of errors.[26] Patient safety, along with an agenda focused on training to prevent errors, and research activities and lessons learned from aviation and occupational health led to development of the Center for Patient Safety within the AHRQ.[27] Quality and safety are positioned together to prevent and report errors, and include topics such as communication, safety culture, and education, and acknowledge the human factors in making mistakes.[27]

Pediatric Quality Metrics and Indicators

Pediatric quality metrics and indicators evolved from adult measures; however, children represent a much smaller population and a much higher risk category, especially when care is based on size, body weight, and management strategies that may not be supported with appropriate research.[28,29] Initial efforts at identifying benchmarks and quality indicators for children began with the Children's Health Insurance Program Reauthorization Act (CHIPRA) in 2009, which introduced the core set of quality measures for children in Medicaid and the Children's Health Insurance Program (CHIP).[28] In 2011, the AHRQ and the CMS initiated the Pediatric Quality Measures Program, including a group of 7 centers of excellence that were asked to develop measures for various aspects of pediatric care.[30] The CHIPRA, along with the CMS, developed the first core pediatric set; the Child Core Set of Health Care Quality Measures.[30] **Table 1** lists highlights of the newest set (2018), which includes 26 measures within 6 areas.[31] Current quality core measures for Medicaid include aspects of preventative care, including weight and nutrition counseling; well child visits at specified intervals; and adolescent screening for mental health problems, sexually transmitted infection, and contraceptive management.[31] Asthma management, dental care, and monitoring of central line–associated bloodstream infections (CLABSIs) in hospital care are other

Table 1
Selections of 2018 core set of children's health care quality measures for Medicaid and the Children's Health Insurance Program

Measure Steward	Measure Name
Primary Care Access and Preventive Care	
NCQA	Chlamydia screening in women ages 16–21 y
NCQA	Childhood immunization status
CMS	Screening for depression and follow-up plan
NCQA	Children and adolescents' access to primary care practitioners
Maternal and Perinatal Health	
CDC	Pediatric central line–associated bloodstream infections
CDC	Audiological diagnosis ≤3 mo of age
CDC	Live births weighing <2500 g
Care of Acute and Chronic Conditions	
NCQA	Asthma medication ratio: ages 5–18 y
NCQA	Ambulatory care: emergency department visits
Behavioral Health	
NCQA	Follow-up care for children prescribed attention-deficit or hyperactivity disorder medication
NCQA	Follow-up after hospitalization for mental illness
NCQA	Use of multiple concurrent antipsychotics in children and adolescents
Dental and Oral Health Services	
CMS	Percentage of eligible children who received preventive dental services
Experience of Care	
NCQA	Consumer Assessment of Healthcare Providers and Systems (CAHPS) health plan survey 5.0 Child version, including Medicaid and children with chronic conditions supplemental items

Abbreviations: CDC, centers for disease control and prevention; NCQA, national committee for quality assurance.
Data from 2018 Core set of children's health care quality measures for Medicaid and CHIP. Available at: https://www.medicaid.gov/medicaid/quality-of-care/downloads/performance-measurement/2018-child-core-set.pdf. Accessed October 1, 2018.

measures in this list.[31] The *Healthcare Effectiveness Data and Information Set* (*HEDIS*) presents health care performance measures, including adult and pediatric criteria. Child and adolescent immunization rates, follow-up for children with mental and behavioral diagnoses, and weight management are some of the benchmarks and threshold measures published by this organization.[32] Despite outlined quality metrics, however, determining pediatric quality indicators continues to represent challenges highlighted in the literature that are based on the 4 Ds: (1) differential epidemiology, acknowledging that children are healthy and seldom have multiple health care problems; (2) dependence on adults for financial support; (3) demographics as childhood age ranges, representing poverty and racial diversity; and (4) development that is constantly changing.[33,34] Pediatric quality indicators continue to evolve and challenges exist in identifying the most important of these based on safety, outcomes, and financial implications.

PEDIATRIC QUALITY METRICS

Children are basically healthy and only a small portion experience severe, chronic illnesses or complex health problems, so there are not as many essential metrics as those used for adults. Pediatric measures are focused on underuse of services, especially in primary care.[28] Many metrics address preventative care in the outpatient arena and many concepts can be easily measured and published, especially with the use of descriptive data. Examples of quality outcomes in the outpatient areas include documentation of immunization rates, attendance at well child visits, and rates of referral to urgent or emergent care.[31] This information is easy to obtain within electronic health records and is collected by many insurance providers. Difficult pediatric data to obtain include coordination of care for children with complex illness, mental health referrals and care, education and support for children who are obese, and monitoring of care for children with other chronic illness.[32] Quality improvement in pediatric health care originates from adult foci; however, pediatric illness varies greatly from that of adults, so domains must feature those concerns of pediatric developmental care along with specific pediatric illness. Since the inception of adult measures in the early 1990s, pediatric measures have been developed and are growing dramatically with objectives focused on providers, payers, institutions, and patients.

Indicators or metrics in pediatric health care quality are relatively new concepts but very important because health care accuracy is imperative. Today's technology-driven environment places children at much higher risk for medical errors and poor outcomes, sometimes simply based on physiologic parameters such as weight, developmental level, and dependency on others for care and treatment.[33] Current pediatric quality indicators have been developed and validated with most implemented by the AHRQ and the CMS, in response to the CHIPRA.[26] Quality measures include those targeted at providers, which are aimed at primary care goals or preventative services, and those that are disease-specific or condition-specific, which are related to diagnostic studies, hospital-based outcomes, or systems of care such as nursing.[27] In addition to the CMS and the AHRQ, other organizations, such as the Children's Hospital Association, the Centers for Disease Control, the AAP, and the American Medical Association, are national organizations that have been responsible for introducing, reviewing, endorsing, or studying pediatric quality measures. House and colleagues[30] (2017) published a collection of identified and classified pediatric quality measures, based on relevance, separated by system or process, and then based on content. Despite the number of quality measures already in place, results also indicate underuse of health care services and continued gaps, including clinical processes such as care of medically complex children, antibiotic stewardship, and avoiding the use of cough and cold preparations in young children. The length of time it takes to apply research to practice; limited collaborative, multicenter QI initiatives; and lack of financial and other resource support are larger, system-based gaps.[28] Another study of interest used a national database of children from 3974 hospitals and reviewed inpatient pediatric quality performance, attempting to identify hospitals with care that is worse than average, which is another method to measure outcomes, offering information for both consumers and payers.[35]

BENCHMARKING IN PEDIATRICS

Because quality measures or indicators are evidence-based and incorporate research activities, expert opinion, and evaluation by national organizations, it is important that measures include multihospital sites and large numbers of patients. Benchmarking is a function that measures large-volume performance tracked over time, measuring an institution's success or failure by comparing specific processes internally, between similar or competitive organizations, and within the health care industry at large.[36] Benchmarking has been used in other industries for much longer than in health care, and it poses opportunities for strategic planning, innovation, and creativity to improve internal processes. Four types of benchmarking have been defined: internal, competitive, functional, and strategic. Internal benchmarking compares performance over time within the organization. Competitive benchmarking compares outcomes with similar organizations. Functional and strategic benchmarking are similar concepts that allow alignment with other organizations to share data or partner to improve performance scores.[35]

Examples of benchmarking in pediatrics include data related to hospital-acquired infections, hospital readmission, asthma and diabetes admission rates, cancer and surgical success rates, and many others, with an expanding list. Recognition and rapid management of sepsis, especially in children, is a very significant benchmark for acute hospitals and emergency departments. A universal initiative is early recognition and management of sepsis in children. Ames and colleagues (2018) completed a retrospective review of 153 hospitals, evaluating pediatric sepsis encounters for the purpose of benchmarking. Risk-adjusted mortality can be used as a quality metric for benchmarking; however, the results of this study were not able to be used because all of the hospitals were located within a close geographic area, limiting generalizability.[36] Managing sepsis in children, with a goal of 0% mortality, is just 1 of the many benchmarks that require universal prevention initiatives and vigilant data collection.

QUALITY AT NEMOURS ALFRED I. duPont HOSPITAL FOR CHILDREN

Children's hospitals are in primary positions to incorporate quality recommendations and measures within set service lines and specialty areas. The Nemours Al duPont Hospital for Children (AIDHC) is a free-standing children's hospital located in the mid-Atlantic area of the United States, with associated outpatient primary and specialty care practices and 2 ambulatory surgery centers. Nemours services are positioned strategically in 4 states, with the main hospital located in Wilmington, Delaware. The Nemours AIDHC is part of a large children's health care system with tertiary, specialty, and primary locations also in Florida. The Nemours system publishes quality metrics in regard to specialty services and benchmarked data. This information is available for patients, families, and the general public. **Table 2** displays some of these data.

Table 2
Pediatric benchmarks and Nemours AI duPont Hospital for Children

	National Pediatric Benchmark	Nemours
Inpatient		
Pediatric Intensive Care Unit Central Venous Line (CVL) Infection Rate	0.62 infections/1000 CVL[a]	3 infections/4806 CVL
Catheter-Associated Urinary Tract Infections	0.37 infections/1000 catheter days[b]	0.5 infections/1347 catheter days
90-d Readmission Rate for Diabetic Ketoacidosis	As high as 10%[c]	<5%
Preventing Emesis After Surgery	4.8%[d]	1.8%
Preventing Postoperative Hypothermia	4.8%[d]	3.2%
Outpatient		
Avoiding Antibiotic Prescriptions for Upper Respiratory Infection	98%[e]	97%
Rates of Children Fully Immunized by age 36 mo	72%[f]	89%
Screening for Chlamydia in Sexually Active Teen Girls	54.6%[g]	79.5%
Percent of Children with Sore Throats Given Antibiotics Only After Positive Tests for Strep Throat	70%–80%[h]	80%

[a] Children's Hospitals' Solutions for Patient Safety Network for 2016 for central line–associated bloodstream infections in pediatric intensive care units.[52]
[b] Childrens' Hospital's Solutions for Patient Safety Network; 2016 for catheter-associated urinary tract infections.[53]
[c] Current State of Type I Diabetes (TID) Treatment in the US: Updated by the TID Exchange Clinic Registry. 38:2015.[54]
[d] National Benchmark for Anesthesiology. Anesthesia Quality Institute's National Clinical Outcomes Registry (2014).[55]
[e] Guidelines by the AAP Recommendation for Managing Common Colds.[56]
[f] Centers for Disease Control and Prevention, National Center for Health Statistics, 2017.[57]
[g] AHRQ Healthcare effectiveness data and information set (HEDIS) pediatric healthcare performance measures website, 2016.[32]
[h] Antibiotic Prescribing and Use in Doctor's Offices, CDC, 2017.[58]

The Wilmington hospital is also engaged in biomedical research activities with focus on asthma, cystic fibrosis, cancer markers and therapeutics, diabetes, and obesity, as well as neurodevelopmental and musculoskeletal diseases. Research in nursing and within interprofessional teams, along with quality improvement initiatives, rank high in maintaining a competitive, state-of-the-art health care program for children. Nemours is most interested in providing family-centered quality care for all children who reside within local areas, as well as offering care to children who live outside the United States.

Strong interprofessional family-focused health care, continuous QI, and research activities form the basis of quality at Nemours. Outcomes data, published by the *US News and World Report*, ranks children's hospitals annually. In the 2018 to 2019 edition, pediatric hospitals were rated in 12 system-based areas of care. Nemours consistently received excellent scores in nursing care, clinical support, commitment to quality improvement, and patient support; providing help for families and enlisting families in structuring care.[37] To sustain their mission, Nemours also provides care to children from outside of the United States, offering them medical and surgical services that may not be available where they live. Nemours values include building and sustaining a culture of trust, and maintaining a continuous journey to provide the best quality, state-of-the-art, and financially feasible health care for children. Nemours associates aim to provide care for every child as if they were their own. Quality and value provide structure for maintaining the mission and insuring ongoing evaluation.

Value-Based Contracts

A first venture into value-based contracting, Nemours partnered with Aetna Health Insurance for a 3-year agreement to establish targets for quality metrics in their physician practice and hospital operations at the AIDHC. Measures for the hospital were divided into 3 categories: efficiency measures, timely and effective care measures, and national program measures.

Targets for efficiency measures were constructed using national claims data from Aetna. Examples of targets in this category included 30-day readmission rate, average length of stay, and adverse events. Measures for the timely and effective care category were based on established quality indicators from the CMS and included infections associated with hospital or health care workers, such as CLABSI, catheter-associated urinary tract infection (CAUTI), and methicillin-resistant *Staphylococcus aureus* infection. National program measures were based on Nemours' participation with a public reporting program, which provides information to the public about hospital outcomes that is readily available for consumers. Nemours participates with the Leapfrog Group, which describes itself as "a nonprofit watchdog organization that serves as a voice for health care purchasers, using their collective influence to foster positive change in U.S. health care."[38] Targets in the national program measures categories included reporting to the Leapfrog Group on computerized physician order entry (prevention of medication errors), appropriate intensive care unit (ICU) staffing, and managing serious errors.

In physician practice, which includes primary care nurse practitioners, examples of measures included well-child visits for children aged 3 to 6 years, immunization targets for adolescent patients, and hemoglobin A1c testing for pediatric patients with diabetes. Nemours and Aetna selected a 24 pediatric indicators and established targets for each indicator. During the first year of the agreement, Nemours met 23 of the 24 targets in quality, the single exception was a physician network participation measure.

The partnership between Aetna and Nemours serves as an example of collaboration between the payer and the health system that focuses on improving the quality of care provided to the children served by both organizations, reducing cost expenditures, and expanding the safe delivery of care. According to Porter and Lee[39] (2013), value-based care is the heart of health care transformation.[40,41] In this payer–service provider collaboration, quality and value are forefront in maintaining the health of children.

Volume

Another monitor for quality is volume, as defined by the number of times a medical or surgical procedure is completed successfully within an institution and illustrated at Nemours through success of the cardiac surgery program. This surgical team has a zero rate of mortality for Norwood, arterial switch, tetralogy of Fallot, and truncus arteriosus procedures compared with national benchmarks from the Society for Thoracic Surgery's congenital heart disease database.[42] Team care provided by nurse practitioners who manage patients in the cardiac ICU and stepdown unit 24 hours a day and skilled bedside nurses, along with the cardiac surgeons, fellows, respiratory care providers, and other professionals, accounts for this successful program.

Infection Prevention

The inpatient data on quality, demonstrated through infection prevention, at Nemours suggest infection rates lower than the benchmarks. The AAP published data collected between 2007 and 2012 from 173 pediatric hospital neonatal ICUs and pediatric ICUs in the United States.[43] During this time, the national CAUTI rate remained static. The national benchmark for hospital-acquired CAUTI was 1.3 per 1000 catheter days. At Nemours, the 2016 rate was 0.5 per 1347 catheter days. Of note, 1 CAUTI can cost the hospital between $911 and $3,824, which among the lowest costs for hospital-acquired infection.[44]

Patient-Centered Medical Home

Another example of pediatric quality is through the Nemours outpatient primary care practices, which are all credentialed as patient-centered medical homes, a designation that aligns patients with providers as partners in care. Coordinated care, enhanced technology, and teamwork are concepts of the medical home philosophy. The National Committee for Quality Assurance has awarded all of the Nemours' Delaware primary care practices level 3 recognition, which is the highest designation achievable through this organization.[45] Patients attending these practices receive improved continuity of care with consistent providers, communication live and through electronic health records with patient compliance with illnesses, such as asthma; and decreased waiting times, among other requirements for certification. Telehealth eliminates the walls of the health care practices, providing opportunities for care outside of the traditional office model.

This Delaware children's hospital publishes care benchmarks for pediatric specialty services comparing results with national averages. Within the outpatient areas of the hospital, which include primary care offices, screening for chlamydia in sexually active adolescent and teen patients is at 79.5% compared with the benchmark rate of 52%. Immunization rates are at 89%, greater than the national rate of 72% (see **Table 2**).

Hospital Readmission Rates

Quality is also maintained through continuous improvement (CI) in this institution in which the LEAN method (principles to assist in solving problems) is used.[46] LEAN thinking is based on the Toyota value and eliminating waste. An example of the CI process to improve quality, reduce waste in time, and use nursing and APN expertise occurred on a short-stay unit where a new streamlined 24-bed short-stay inpatient care model was developed that addresses efficacy and quality outcomes with decreased hospital readmission rates. This new patient care model incorporates an APN-led medical team, in which the interprofessional team huddles determine patient discharge needs, while nurses expedite transfers from the emergency department, postanesthesia care unit, or other inpatient areas by physically going to the transferring area, evaluating, and accompanying the patient to the unit for admission. Clinical pathways were designed and are used to address patient management by diagnosis. With expedited admission and discharge criteria, the length of stay has decreased and there remains an objective transfer to the floor time of less than 60 minutes.

On-Call Costs

Members of the department of nursing, independently and in collaboration with other disciplines, identify clinical problems, create research and EBP questions, and complete projects aimed at improving care at the bedside. An administrative nurse researcher and a research fellowship program in which EBP and research methodology are taught support these endeavors. One such project was completed in the pediatric sedation suite where baseline data indicated costs for on-call nursing services had quadrupled between 2013 and 2016. Through rapid process improvement methods, nurse team leaders created and tested an algorithm to improve communication and streamlined processes for case preparation, which resulted in greater than $20,000 reduction in costs for 2018. Reviewing current practices of time spent per nurse in arranging cases from home, developing a new method for physicians to collaborate with nursing to identify patient priority level, along with creation of order sets designed to standardize procedures, formed the basic features of this algorithm.

Documentation Improvement

Another interprofessional project with a focus on safety and quality was an analysis of recorded patient heights and weights, an intervention to improve documentation and a current data collection to monitor success. Following implementation of interventions, nurses, clinical dieticians, physicians, and pharmacists continue to evaluate discrepancies in patient-recorded anthropometrics and the relationship to medication errors and appropriate nutrition consults. This seemingly simple project assists in improving quality without hospital costs beyond education and purchasing new scales.

PATIENT-FOCUSED HEALTH CARE

One of the newest national initiatives in relation to pediatric quality is a focus on patient involvement in health care and health care reform, which is also 1 of the 6 NAM domains of patient-centered care.[47] Customized patient care, allowing for patient control, as well as transparency and open information sharing, is part of this design. Even in pediatrics, methods to address and evaluate the presence of patients and families in health care decision-making are still rudimentary. Surveys are used by most health care institutions to obtain patient evaluation of recent care and to allow patients and families an opportunity to talk about their experiences. The hospital Consumer Assessment of Healthcare Providers and Systems (CAHPS) was initially designed for adult patient responses but has expanded to include a pediatric format.[48] The development, field testing, and validation of the pediatric CAHPS survey, published in *Pediatrics* (2015), was an extensive scientific endeavor, funded by the CMS and the AHRQ through the Pediatric Quality Measures Program.[48] Parent focus groups and individual parent interviews were part of the tool development. The AHRQ has published compiled response data from CAHPS for the years 2007 to 2017 for children with Medicaid and the CHIP. From this, 2017 composite responses indicated the highest scores for CHIP and Medicaid were in the areas of how well doctors communicate, rating of personal doctor, and getting care quickly.[49] Determining quality or value-based care through survey modalities is among the first opportunities for parents and families to be involved in evaluation of care.

Advisory Councils

Other avenues for parent participation in pediatric quality include inviting parents to be part of hospital boards, become policy advocates, and participate in facility design decision-making. At Nemours, parents and families are an integral part of care for children. The hospital hosts a Family Advisory Council composed of members of the community, primarily parents, who provide family feedback to improve processes, advocate for change, and become involved in decision-making. The Youth Advisory

Council is composed of children between the ages of 8 and 17 years, who also weigh in on improving the experiences of children who are patients at Nemours. The Family as Faculty program provides opportunities for parents to share their expertise in caring for their children throughout illness because parents are knowledgeable and expert resources in their child's illness. The practice of pediatrics has always been family-focused; however, these endeavors open communication and allow family perspectives to improve care for children.

SUMMARY OR DISCUSSION

Health care in the United States continues to evolve, with an overall goal of patient-focused, patient-informed, and patient-involved care; however, obstacles and barriers still persist that preclude evidence from being applied to practice and timing is still not ideal. Health care in the United States carries a very high cost compared with other well-developed countries and costs are expected to increase annually. It is most important now to guarantee that hospitals adapt their practice to benchmarks and use high-volume activities to maximize quality and safety.

Nurses represent the largest group of health care providers in the United States, are educated in EBP, and have an important impact on patient quality and safety, especially in pediatric hospitals. The NAM's 2010 report, *The Future of Nursing: Leading Change, Advancing Health*, states that nurses need to practice to their fullest extent of education and training, achieve higher levels of education, and be full partners with MDs and other health care professionals.[4] Patient care leaders need to be positioned to support clinical nurses in endeavors to address quality, create new benchmarks, and improve patient safety through quality and CI projects and processes. Most important is that evidence obtained by nurses be disseminated. Nemours' nurses have accomplished improvements in many arenas of nursing care and continue to be engaged in these endeavors. Research and quality improvement projects have changed practice within this institution, and can be used as evidence of success for other children's hospitals. Coaching nurses to prepare and publish articles is very important but requires time and expertise from experienced coaches and leaders.[50] Children's hospital nursing departments have an opportunity to collaborate with interprofessional colleagues in research and evidence data collection within their own hospital systems and among networks of children's hospitals, such as the Children's Hospital Association. Solutions for Patient Safety is a network of children's hospitals, including Nemours, and has joined forces to decrease the rates of hospital-acquired conditions, and promote patient safety and quality through transparency and a culture in which nurses can feel free to communicate concerns.[51]

Finally, it can take at least 17 years for health care research to be translated into practice, which is too long, essentially an entire childhood. Innovation, participation in quality initiatives, and benchmarking are important initiatives for nursing departments. Nurses and families are large-volume stakeholders in health care with endless opportunities to promote quality outcomes and limit errors in the campaign of pediatric care.

REFERENCES

1. Google dictionary, definition of quality website. Available at: https://www.google.com/search?q=definitiion+of+quality&rls=com.microsoft:en-US&ie=UTF-8&oe=UTF-8&startIndex=&startPage=1&safe=strict&gws_rd=ssl#spf=1538060013239. Accessed June 14, 2018.

2. World Health Organization: maternal, newborn, child and adolescent health. Standards for improving the quality of care for children and young adolescents in health facilities website. Available at: http://www.who.int/maternal_child_adolescent/documents/quality-standards-child-adolescent/en/. Accessed June 25, 2018.
3. Institute of Medicine of the National Academies. Crossing the quality chasm: a new health system for the 21st century website. 2001. Available at: http://www.nationalacademies.org/hmd/~/media/Files/Report%20Files/2001/Crossing-the-Quality-Chasm/Quality%20Chasm%202001%20%20report%20brief.pdf. Accessed June 14, 2018.
4. Institute of Medicine of the National Academies, Committee on the Robert Wood Johnson Foundation Initiative on the Future of Nursing, at the Institute of Medicine. The future of nursing: leading change, advancing health website. 2010. Available at: https://www.nap.edu/read/12956/chapter/1. Accessed June 14, 2018.
5. Agency for Healthcare Research and Quality. National healthcare quality and disparities report website. 2018. Available at: https://www.ahrq.gov/research/findings/nhqrdr/index.html. Accessed September 25, 2018.
6. Bonow RO, Masoudi JS, Rumsfeld ED, et al. ACC/AHA classification of care metrics: performance measures and quality metrics: a report of the American College of Cardiology/American Heart Association task force on performance measures. Circulation 2008;118(24):2662–6.
7. Ayanian JZ, Markel H. Donabedian's lasting framework for health care quality. N Engl J Med 2016;375(3):205–7.
8. National Quality Forum: NQF's work in quality measurement website. Available at: http://www.qualityforum.org/about_nqf/work_in_quality_measurement/. Accessed September 28, 2018.
9. Centers for Medicare and Medicaid Services website. Available at: CMS.gov https://www.cms.gov/Medicare/Quality-Initiatives-Patient-Assessment-Instruments/QualityMeasures/index.html. Accessed August 3, 2018.
10. The Centers for Medicaid and Medicare Services. Integrated care for kids model; fact sheet 2018. Available at: https://www.cms.gov/newsroom/fact-sheets/integrated-care-kids-inck-model. Accessed October 1, 2018.
11. Centers for Medicare and Medicaid Services. Quality measures development overview. Available at: https://www.cms.gov/medicare/quality-initiatives-patient-assessment-instruments/qualityinitiativesgeninfo/downloads/qualitymeasures developmentoverview.pdf. Accessed March 5, 2019.
12. American Academy of Pediatrics. Quality improvement website. 2018. Available at: https://www.aap.org/en-us/professional-resources/quality-improvement/Pages/default.aspx. Accessed September 12, 2018.
13. American Academy of Pediatrics Steering Committee on Quality Improvement and Management, American Academy of Pediatrics Committee on Practice and Ambulatory Medicine. Principles for the development and use of quality measures. Pediatrics 2008;121(2):411–8.
14. National quality forum website. Available at: http://www.qualityforum.org/Show_Content.aspx?id=119. Accessed September 26, 2018.
15. Mainz J. Defining and classifying clinical indicators for quality improvement. Int J Qual Health Care 2003;15(6):523–30.
16. AHRQ types of quality measures website. 2015. Available at: https://www.ahrq.gov/professionals/quality-patient-safety/talkingquality/create/types.html. Accessed September 25, 2018.

17. Mackey A, Bassendowski S. The history of evidence-based practice in nursing education and practice. J Prof Nurs 2017;33(1):51–5.
18. Montalvo I. The National Database of Nursing Quality Indicators (NDNQI). American Nurses Association OJIN 2007;12(3). Available at: http://ojin.nursingworld.org/MainMenuCategories/ANAMarketplace/ANAPeriodicals/OJIN/TableofContents/Volume122007/No3Sept07/NursingQualityIndicators.html. Accessed September 29, 2018.
19. McDonald KM. Approach to improving quality: the role of quality measurement and a case study of the Agency for Healthcare Research and Quality pediatric quality indicators. Pediatr Clin North Am 2009;56:815–29.
20. Brower EJ, Nemec R. Origins of evidence based practice and what it means for nurses. Int J Childbirth Educ 2017;32(2):14–8.
21. Sackett DL, Rosenberg WM, Gray M, et al. Evidence based medicine: what it is and what it isn't. BMJ 1996;312(7023):71–2.
22. Melnyk BM, Gallagher-Ford L, Long EL, et al. The establishment of evidence-based competencies for practicing registered nurses and advanced practice nurses in real-world clinical settings: proficiencies to improve healthcare quality, reliability, patient outcomes and cost. Worldviews Evid Based Nurs 2014;11(1):5–15.
23. QSEN Institute. Frances Payne Bolton School of Nursing, Case Western University. Quality and safety education for nurses website. 2012. Available at: http://www.qsen.org/competencies/. Accessed September 26, 2018.
24. American Association of Critical Care Nurses. AACN synergy model for patient care website. Available at: https://www.aacn.org/nursing-excellence/aacn-standards/synergy-model. n.d. Accessed September 26, 2018.
25. Hardin SR, Kaplow R. Synergy for clinical excellence. Burlington (MA): Jones and Bartlett Learning; 2017.
26. Institute of Medicine of the National Academies. To err is human: building a safer health system. 1999. Available at: http://www.nationalacademies.org/hmd/~/media/Files/Report%20Files/1999/To-Err-is-Human/To%20Err%20is%20Human%201999%20%20report%20brief.pdf. Accessed September 26, 2018.
27. AHRQ patient safety network: center for patient safety website. 2018. Available at: https://psnet.ahrq.gov/resources/resource/2342/center-for-patient-safety. Accessed September 26, 2018.
28. Schwartz SP, Rehder KJ. Quality improvement in pediatrics: past, present and future. Pediatr Res 2017;81(1):156–61.
29. Dougherty D, Mistry KB, Llanos K, et al. An AHRQ and CMS perspective on the pediatric quality measures program. Acad Pediatr 2014;14:S17–8.
30. House SA, Coon ER, Schroeder AR, et al. Categorization of national pediatric quality measures. Pediatrics 2017;139(4):1–8.
31. Child core health care quality measurement set website. 2018. Available at: https://www.medicaid.gov/federal-policy-guidance/downloads/cib111417.pdf. Accessed June 30, 2018.
32. AHRQ Healthcare effectiveness data and information set (HEDIS) pediatric healthcare performance measures website. 2016. Available at: https://www.ncqa.org/hedis/. Accessed September 26, 2018.
33. Simpson L, Dougherty D, Krause D, et al. Measuring children's health care quality. Am J Med Qual 2007;22(2):80–4.
34. Mangione-Smith R. The challenges of addressing pediatric quality measurement gaps. Pediatrics 2017;139(4):1–2.

35. Berry JG, Zaslavsky AM, Toomey SL, et al. Recognizing differences in hospital quality performance for pediatric inpatient care. Pediatrics 2015;136(2):251–62.
36. Kumar B. Patient safety and quality metrics in pediatric hospital medicine. Pediatr Clin North Am 2016;63:283–91.
37. Fibuch E, Van Way CW. Benchmarking's role in driving performance. Physician Exec 2013;39:28–32.
38. The Leapfrog Group website. 2018. Available at: http://www.leapfroggroup.org/ratings-reports. Accessed September 26, 2018.
39. Porter ME, Lee TH. The strategy that will fix health care. HRB 2013.
40. Ames SG, Davis BS, Angus DC, et al. Hospital variation in risk-adjusted pediatric sepsis mortality. Pediatr Crit Care Med 2018;19(5):390–6.
41. Best children's hospitals 2018-2019. US News and World Report. Available at: https://www.usnews.com/info/blogs/press-room/articles/2018-06-26/us-news-announces-the-2018-2019-best-childrens-hospitals. Accessed September 26, 2018.
42. Society for Thoracic Surgery. Congenital heart surgery database. Spring; 2018. Available at: https://www.sts.org/registries-research-center/sts-national-database/sts-congenital-heart-surgery-database. Accessed September 26, 2018.
43. Patrick SW, Kawai AT, Kleinman K, et al. Healthcare associated infections among critically ill children in the US, 2007-2012. Pediatrics 2014;134(4):1–8.
44. Kennedy EH, Greene MT, Saint S. Estimating hospital costs of catheter associated urinary tract infections. J Hosp Med 2013;8(9):519–22.
45. National Committee for Quality Assurance. Patient-centered medical home. 2018. Available at: https://www.ncqa.org/programs/health-care-providers-practices/patient-centered-medical-home-pcmh/. Accessed September 27, 2018.
46. Womack JP, Byme AP, Flume OJ, et al. Going Lean in health care: executive summary. Institute for Healthcare Improvement; 2005. NCQA Measuring Quality Improving Health care. Patient-Centered Medical Home Recognition. Available at: www.ncqa.org/programs/recognition/practices/patient-centered-medical-home-pcmh. Accessed September 25, 2018.
47. Agency for Healthcare Research and Quality. The six domains of healthcare quality website. 2015. Available at: https://www.ahrq.gov/professionals/quality-patient-safety/talkingquality/create/sixdomains.html. Accessed September 27, 2018.
48. Toomey SA, Zaslavsky AM, Elliott MN, et al. The development of a pediatric inpatient experience of care measure: child HCAHPS. Pediatrics 2015;136(2):360–9.
49. Agency for Healthcare Research and Quality. Health plan survey chartbook. 2017. Available at: https://www.ahrq.gov/cahps/cahps-database/comparative-data/2017-health-plan-chartbook/executive-summary.html. Accessed November 7, 2018.
50. Kooker BM, Latimer R, Mark DD. Successfully coaching nursing staff to publish outcomes. J Nurs Adm 2015;43(12):636–41.
51. Butler GA, Hupp DS. Pediatric quality and safety: a nursing perspective. Pediatr Clin North Am 2016;63:329–39.
52. Children's Hospitals' solutions for patient safety network for 2016 for central line-associated bloodstream infections in pediatric intensive care units. SPS Prevention Bundles. https://www.solutionsforpatientsafety.org/wp-content/SPS-Prevention-Bundles.pdf. Accessed March 5, 2019.
53. Childen's hospitals' solutions for patient safety network; 2016 for catheter-associated urinary tract infections. https://www.solutionsforpatientsafety.org/wp-content/SPS-Prevention-Bundles.pdf. Accessed March 5, 2019.

54. Miller KM, Foster NC, Beck RW, et al. Current state of type 1 diabetes treatment in the US: Updated data from the T1D Exchange Clinic Registry. American Diabetes Association: Diabetes Care 2015;38(6):971–8. Available at: Care. diabetesjournals.org/content/38/6/971. Accessed March 5, 2019.
55. National Benchmark for Anesthesiology. Anesthesia Quality Institute, National Anesthesia Clinical Outcomes Registry (NACOR). Available at: www.aqihq.org/introduction-to-nacor.aspx. Accessed March 5, 2019
56. Choosing Wisely: American Academy of Pediatrics. Ten things physicians and patients should question. 2018. Available at: www.choosingwisely.org/societies/american-academy-of-pediatrics/. Accessed March 5, 2019.
57. Centers for Disease Control and Prevention. National Center for Health Statistics: Immunization. 2017. Available at: https//www.cdc.gov/nchs/fastats/immunize.htm. Accessed March 5, 2019.
58. Centers for Disease Control and Prevention Antibiotic Prescribing and Use in Doctor's Offices. 2017. Available at: https://www.cdc.org/antibiotic-use/community/index.html. Accessed March 5, 2019.

Geriatric Trends Facing Nursing with the Growing Aging

Jolie Harris, DNS, RN

KEYWORDS

• Aging population • Frailty • Social determinants • Interdisciplinary syndrome care

KEY POINTS

- Health care systems in the United States will be impacted by the growing elderly population with longer life expectancy, which is expected to exceed 84 million by 2050.
- This longevity has resulted in more complex multiple chronic conditions that no longer can be managed under current models.
- Frailty has been described as the new tsunami or catastrophe similar to the prevalence of Alzheimer's disease and yet is significantly behind in understanding this complex syndrome.
- Providers are challenged to develop expertise in the assessment, treatment, and evaluation of these challenging geriatric syndromes.
- Interprofessional care models in place of single disease care models will be essential to achieve positive outcomes. Advanced practice nurses are in a strong position to facilitate change and meet the needs of this growing population.

INTRODUCTION

The Gerontological Society of America (GSA) was established in 1945 with a focus on promotion of research in aging and a current membership of more than 5,000 professionals representing a broad range of disciplines.[1] The mission of the society is to promote multidisciplinary and interdisciplinary research in aging, disseminate research, and support aging education, including higher education.[1] In 2017 GSA provided a series of *Trend Reports in Aging* accompanied by a webinar moderated by Dr Resnick, 2017 GSA president.[2–6] The webinar included the 4 section chairs to discuss key topics provided in their respective trend reports and open discussion on topics of prime importance for the future of aging services. The 4 sections and respective chairs included the Health Sciences Section (Dr Griebling), the Social Research, Policy and Practice Section (Ms Sykes), the Behavioral and Social Sciences Section (Dr Pillemer),

Disclosure: The author has nothing to disclose.
LSUHSC New Orleans, 1900 Gravier Street, New Orleans, LA 70112, USA
E-mail address: Jharr9@lsuhsc.edu

and the Biological Sciences Section (Dr Zugich). The GSA followed these initial trend reports with a report in 2018 from 2 of the sections (Social Research and Policy and Health Sciences).[2,7] Key topics from these trend reports and webinar are explored in the areas of population growth, frailty, interdisciplinary syndrome care, social determinants of health, and provider availability as they relate to the growing elderly population, outcomes, and the role of the nurse. Further exploration of reimbursement and the financial impact in supporting these initiatives is also addressed.

POPULATION GROWTH

A discussion related to the aging population necessitates a review of the anticipated growth of the elderly population and interrelated importance to each of the key issues to be addressed. By 2050, the population of those age 65 and older in the United States will be nearly 84 million, almost double the population in 2012 with surviving Baby Boomers all over the age of 85.[8] The growth of the oldest old (age $\geq$85 years) is projected to double by 2036 and triple by 2049[8] (**Figs. 1** and **2**). Life expectancy has improved over the past 30 years. In 1972, the average life expectancy at age 65 was 15.2 years (to age 80.2); by 2010, the average life expectancy at age 65 had increased by 4 years to 19.1 years (to age 84.2).[8] There will be a greater percent of females in the older age groups, especially in 85 years and over (>60%) who are more likely to be widowed.[8] The population will become more ethnically and racially diverse, with a growing Hispanic proportion.[8]

After the Baby Boomer generation, birth rates began to decrease, which has resulted in lower ratios of working-age population, defined as ages 18 to 64 years, in proportion to the older population.[8] In 2010, there were 21 elderly for every 100 adults in the working age contrasted with the projection in 2050 of 36 elderly for every 100 working-age adults[8] (**Fig. 3**). There will be less working population to support the

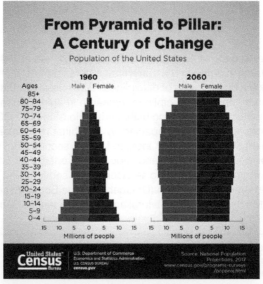

Fig. 1. Population change in the United States. (*From* United States Census Bureau. Pyramid to pillar: a century of change. Available at: https://www.census.gov/library/visualizations/2018/comm/century-of-change.html. Accessed November 9, 2018.)

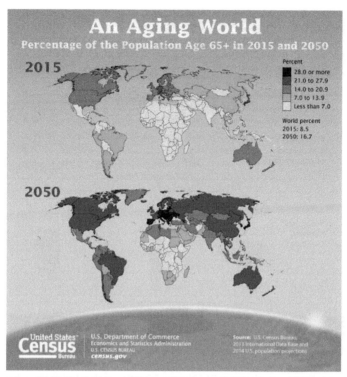

Fig. 2. An aging world. Percentage of the population age 65 years or older in 2015 and 2050. (*From* United States Census Bureau. An aging world. Available at: https://www.census.gov/library/visualizations/2016/comm/cb16-54_aging_world.html. Accessed November 9, 2018.)

ever-increasing volume and needs of the elderly from a support and financial perspective. Ninety percent of the households of those 65 and older receive Social Security and this number increase to as many as 94% for those 85 and older.[9] In 2014, at least one-half of the income for persons 65 and older was received from Social Security.[10] The poverty rate was higher for women, reaching 13% for people who were 85 and older and 18.1% for Hispanics.[9,10] With the population growth, larger shares of total resources may be spent on health care and caregiving in the future.

The growth of the elderly population, in the United States and globally, has been a topic of discussion for years as experts outlined the staggering numbers from the Baby Boomer generation to move into the over 65 classification. Combined with the increasing numbers of the older population is the extended life expectancy (higher with females) and shift in racial and ethnic composition to a higher percentage of non-white population and an increase in Hispanic origin (5-fold)[8] (**Fig. 4**). Along with this shift is the decreased growth rate of the post-Baby Boomer generation to support the needs of the growing elderly population. These challenges are important to be abreast of as we explore key future trends.

FRAILTY

Dr Nikolich-Zugich, chair of the Biological Science Section, Department Chair of the Department of Immunobiology, and Co-Director of the Arizona Center on Aging at the University of Arizona, in identifying 1 of the 3 areas of concern facing the care of

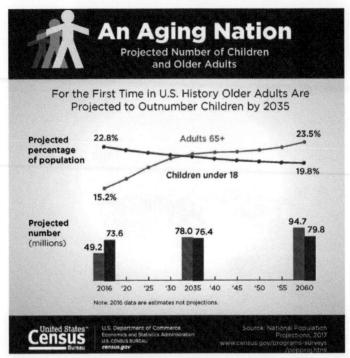

Fig. 3. Aging nation. (*From* United States Census Bureau. An aging nation. Available at: https://www.census.gov/library/visualizations/2018/comm/historic-first.html. Accessed November 9, 2018.)

the aging population, identified frailty. Dr Nikolich-Zugich described this concern as a tsunami or catastrophe similar to the prevalence of Alzheimer's disease.[11] He further explained that the study of frailty is about 30 to 35 years behind Alzheimer's in understanding the syndrome, yet the incidence is similar.[11]

Frailty is a condition "characterized by a decrease of reserves and functions across multiple physiologic systems, responsible for a compromised ability to cope with stressors."[12] The Frailty Index has operationalized frailty by the presence of 3 or more of the following components: unintentional weight loss, fatigue, weakness, decreased walking speed, and low physical activity level.[13] Adverse outcomes, such as death, falls, fractures, and hospitalizations, are associated with those experiencing frailty.[12,14] In a large European study, the prevalence of frailty for those aged 65 and older was 17% and those considered prefrail was as high as 42.3%.[15] Frailty is more common in women and those with a lower socioeconomic status.[15] Considering these factors, the urgency to expand research and understanding of this syndrome supports Dr Nikolich-Zugich's concern as a critical area for focus in caring for the growing aging population. Nurses and advance practice nurses fill a crucial role in gaining expertise in all aspects of this syndrome, from assessment and management to monitoring outcomes.

Dr Nikolich-Zugich described the challenge of conducting research on frailty owing to the difficulty in defining the syndrome and complexity of the syndrome.[11] This finding was supported in the article by Chen and colleagues,[16] who noted the lack of consensus on a single operational definition.[16] There is agreement to define frailty

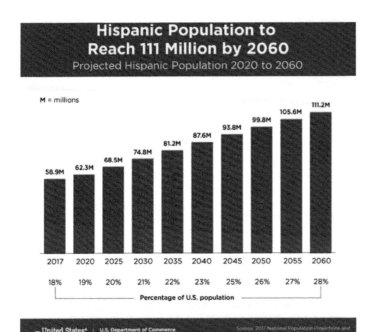

Fig. 4. Shift in the Hispanic population. (*From* United States Census Bureau. Hispanic population to reach 111 million by 2060. Available at: https://www.census.gov/library/visualizations/2018/comm/hispanic-projected-pop.html. Accessed November 9, 2018.)

as a clinical syndrome with increased vulnerability to stressors that lead to negative health outcomes.[16] In lieu of these challenges, research has identified an association of frailty with chronic inflammation and immune activation.[16] More recent studies are exploring biological responses, such as the study by Calvani and colleagues[17] analyzing biomarkers for sarcopenia and physical frailty. The hope is that studies like this will lead to an improved understanding of the pathophysiological pathways of frailty to develop interventions for treatment or monitoring.

From a behavioral science perspective, studies on frailty have been challenging owing to not only ambiguity of the definition, but also to a multitude of measurement instruments.[14] Theou and colleagues[18] in a scoping review on gaps in frailty research identified a number of issues: use of nonfrailty tools to measure frailty; lack of patient-oriented outcomes, such as quality of life; and limited clinical trial studies. From a behavioral and health science standpoint, interventions that have been identified as beneficial are exercise, nutrition, and comprehensive interdisciplinary assessment and treatment.[16] Even with these challenges, studies have grown in recent years with discussions occurring across clinical, social, public health, and research arenas.[14] The study of frailty is not limited to geriatrics or gerontology fields, but has been explored by other disciplines, including emergency medicine, cardiology, orthopedics, oncology, and general medicine.[18] This growing interest signifies the expansive nature of this phenomena.

Chen and colleagues[16] share that frailty may be reversible and, therefore, its recognition and management is essential in slowing progression and preventing disability.[19] de Llano and colleagues,[13] in a study of more than 800 participants 60 years or older, identified the importance of the nurse's role in assessing elders for frailty and implementing individualized care plans to minimize the effects and prevent the consequences of the syndrome. Variables associated with frailty were low education level, obesity, lack of physical activity, cognitive deficit, poor health self-promotion, falls in the prior 12 months, and morbidity.[13] These factors were incorporated in design of the care plan for each participant using a frailty algorithm with a focus on health promotion, prevention, or reversal of frailty and/or rehabilitation. The algorithm classifies the client into 3 levels (nonfrail, prefrail, and frail) with corresponding interventions.[13] Interventions align with the underlying variables, such as education, nutritional assessment and guidance, assessment of muscle strength and exercise prescription, cognitive assessment and stimulation strategies, fall screening and prevention initiatives, and evaluation of the effects of polypharmacy.[13] Whether in a community, acute, or long-term care setting, nurses will be faced with the frailty syndrome and challenged to work with individuals in averting or managing this condition. Using instruments to classify frailty and tools to guide individualized treatment plans are essential to effectively manage this complex syndrome.

Chen and colleagues[20] support the views of Dr Nikolich-Zugich in stating frailty is an "emerging geriatric giant and poses wide-reaching consequences for the individual, family and society in the future." The complexity of this syndrome requires a multifaceted approach from a research and a practice perspective to manage this escalating challenge for the future. The description of the complexity of frailty in understanding the heterogeneous nature of the syndrome leads to the second key trend to explore: interdisciplinary syndrome care.

INTERDISCIPLINARY SYNDROME CARE

Dr Griebling,[6] chair of the Health Science Section, Senior Associate Dean for Medical Education at the University of Kansas School of Medicine, and Faculty Associate in The Landon Center on Aging, discussed in the trend report the challenge to discover ways to provide smarter care by focusing on geriatric syndromes rather than diagnosis-focused care. As described by Dr Griebling,[6] the focus is on treating the whole person instead of an organ system or specialty. In the webinar, Dr Griebling was asked to expand his discussion on syndrome-based care and the hurdles facing the ability to implement this approach.

Dr Griebling described the complexity of geriatric syndromes which typically have multifactorial causes and require various approaches to address the problem.[11] He offered an example in his role as a urologist managing a patient with incontinence and approaching the patient from a diagnosis perspective, dealing strictly with the type of incontinence rather than the larger picture to include possible issues of cognition, mobility limitations, or environmental factors.[11] He stresses in his example, that under syndrome care, the condition is not just limited to the bladder, but other aspects impacting a successful treatment plan.[11] Successful outcomes can only be achieved with a coordinated approach across disciplines, including monitoring multidimensional indicators. In syndrome care, the emphasis is on interdisciplinary care to provide a comprehensive view for planning and treatment.

Geriatric syndromes are characterized as multiple complex health states that cannot be classified into a discrete disease category and tend to occur later in life.[15] The presenting complaint may not reflect the underlying pathologic condition. Acute cognitive decline or falls may be indicative of an underlying condition such as an infection, drug interactions, or environmental factors.[15] Conditions considered to be included in the category of geriatric syndromes are frailty, urinary incontinence, falls, delirium, and pressure ulcers.[15] The coordination of care across disciplines to achieve effective outcomes is limited under the current model of health services delivery.

Hurdles identified by Dr Griebling including the challenge to formulate teams to practice in this manner owing to the individual workload and lack of structures designed to foster interdisciplinary treatment.[11] A second hurdle was financing and reimbursement.[11] The current payment structure is designed by the use of procedural codes and specialized treatment. Dr Griebling described a grant project using an interdisciplinary model in which he participates as a member of a multicenter group via telemedicine to provide group behavioral care for adult patients with incontinence, which allows for economy of scale versus one-on-one care from multiple providers.[11] Examples like the one shared by Dr Griebling provide insight into possible ways to alter practice settings to meet the changing needs of the older population.

The literature supports Dr Griebling's viewpoint. Searle and Rockwood,[21] in describing frailty in the hospital setting, challenge providers to alter their view of the patient. They describe providers who have a primary disease focus and expect patients to present with well-defined problems that can be addressed with a structured course of treatment.[21] Searle and Rockwood[21] refer to this in the following manner: "Disease focused specialist who push on with the only course they know sometimes decry their frail patients as being unsuitable or requiring social support or failing to cope or thrive." Cesari and colleagues[22] echo a similar sentiment in describing the traditional approach of "stand-alone disease medicine" as being out of date in dealing with patients presenting with multiple conditions and syndromes. The risks associated with maintaining the traditional disease state approach include polypharmacy, because the patient is treated for multiple conditions simultaneously and undertreatment or inappropriate treatment of clinical conditions owing to lack of knowledge of the patient or poor understanding of syndrome care.[22] Patients, especially elderly patients, arrive with multiple issues with interacting medical and social etiologies that place them at greater risk for adverse outcomes. Both articles advocate for an approach that views the holistic individual versus a defined disease.

Support was also noted for Dr Griebling's comments in regard to expanding the interdisciplinary team in elder care management. In the discussion presented by Chen and colleagues[20] on the approach to frailty in primary care and the community, the authors point out the importance of a partnership among various health care providers (physician, nurse, social worker, case manager, dietician, allied health staff, exercise trainers, etc), together with the patient, which is needed to achieve significant and sustained improvement. Inzitari and colleagues[19] describe an interventional program focused on managing frailty, including multiple disciplines with a focus on physical exercise, nutritional support, healthy lifestyle education, and polypharmacy adjustments. The study is ongoing, but supports the messages shared by others on the need to shift from disease focused care to multiperspective care eliciting the expertise of a variety of disciplines.

Nurses and advance practice nurses have a significant role in interdisciplinary syndrome care. Hansen and colleagues[23] describe a nurse practitioner–led, interprofessional geriatric clinic operating within a rehabilitation hospital. Included as team members are a social worker and physical and occupational therapists. Referrals are mainly received from primary health care providers for patients displaying an acute change in condition that requires further evaluation from a clinician with geriatric expertise.[23] Both patients and referring practitioners expressed a high level of satisfaction and additional, nonreferred issues were frequently identified during the assessment process.[23]

The Collaboration for Hospitalized Elders Reducing the Impact of Stays in Hospital (CHERISH) is a program under evaluation on nongeriatric hospital units led by a facilitator who possesses skills centered on multidisciplinary team facilitation, geriatric expertise, and the evaluation of cycles of improvement.[24] The outcomes measured include a decrease in geriatric syndromes (delirium, functional decline, falls, pressure injuries, and new incontinence), decreases in length of stay, and decreases in institutional care.[24] Advanced practice nurses are ideally positioned to understand risk factors and geriatric syndromes, translate research into practice, and analyze outcomes. The successful implementation of integrated multidisciplinary programs are often limited by the lack of leadership expertise in the field of geriatric care and treatment.[25] Advance practice nurses can foster the expansion of knowledge and skills central to not only direct care givers, but also decision makers in guiding best practice model development.

Searle and Rockwood[21] summarized the benefit of person-centered health care to center on not only what the patient needs, but what they want, with the goals of better mobility, function, cognition, continence, pain control, and social engagement. To achieve these outcomes, coordination from a myriad of disciplines will be required to provide a unique perspective for overall goal attainment.

As we explore the multimodal, chronic disease processes affecting the elderly, it is important to examine from a broader perspective what information is available to address prevention and screening for high-risk individuals. The third focus area is social determinants of health.

SOCIAL DETERMINANTS OF HEALTH

Ms Sykes, Chair of Social Research, Policy and Practice Section, is retired from her most recent position as Senior Advisor for Aging and Public Health with the Environmental Protection Agency and prior positions as the Associate Director at the Centers for Disease Control and Prevention National Institute for Occupational Safety and Health, and Professional Staff with the US Senate Special Committee on Aging. Sykes identified health inequalities as 1 of her top 3 areas of concern in the future of aging.[11] Sykes shared her views on the social determinants of health and discussed income and health inequalities in the elderly, highlighting the differences as they relate to age and ethnicity.[3] In the report, Trends in Social Research, Policy and Practice,[3] Sykes explains this point in referring to the National Institute on Aging research report on health inequities that noted "Older U.S. racial and ethnic minority populations suffer premature morbidity over the life course, pointing to biological-environmental interactions that hold important implications for understanding mechanisms to explain health disparities." She identified the need to align policy to narrow the gap with the goal to improve care for all people, which can benefit the economic landscape through savings in health care expenditures. Sykes shared data from a report of The Joint Center for Political and Economic Studies, which calculated a savings of $229 billion dollars in the United States from 2003 to 2006 if health inequities had been eliminated.[26]

When viewing the issue of health and disease, society has generally focused on the health sector to address concerns, but as more information is gained on the impact of social determinants on health, the realization occurs that the issue is broader than the health sector alone. The conditions in which one is born, grows, lives, works, and ages are key determinants of health and mostly responsible for health inequities.[27] The distribution of money, power, and resources shape the circumstances of these conditions.[27] The issues must expand to include government, society, local communities, support agencies, and businesses, along with the health care sector to address these challenges.

Reutter and Kushner[28] call nurses to this critical issue in stating, "nursing has a clear mandate to ensure access to health and health-care by providing sensitive empowering care to those experiencing inequities and working to change underlying social conditions that result in and perpetuate health inequities." The call to action includes strengthening the knowledge base on disparities and their effects, providing sensitive and nonjudgmental care, advocacy, and participating in research outlining outcomes supporting the need for change.[28] The authors point out the strong link between nursing, as a caring profession, and social inequities, which are the result of a lack of caring.[28] Nurses, through their daily interactions, witness the effects of health inequities at the individual level and can intervene through planned interventions. Advanced practice nurses and experienced nurses can mentor new nurses through their approach in caring for this population, which often experiences a lack of compassion. From a broader perspective, the authors call for nurses to advocate for change, not just in their own practice settings, but also for improved living and working conditions.[28] An example offered was a group in Canada with a nurse practitioner as one of the founding members with their primary focus on education, outreach to raise awareness of the impact of poverty on health outcomes, advocacy, and research.[28] The evaluation of outcomes as they relate to age, ethnicity, or income can provide insight into establishing specifically designed protocols.

The Commission on Social Determinants of Health included in its final recommendations to expand interdisciplinary research on the social determinants of health to decrease health inequities[29] (**Box 1**). Additionally, the report called for the expanded training of health practitioners to further understand the problem of health inequity, the social determinants, and possible solutions to build public and political awareness.[29] The report notes the limited inclusion of this topic in curriculums and training programs for health professionals, including nurses, and recommends its inclusion at the basic level of education.[29] A greater awareness of health inequities and gender influences on health outcomes is needed to guide practice strategies, including a focus on prevention and health promotion. The report calls for teaching and training materials on the social determinants of health to be accessible through free access sites to facilitate expanded education.[29]

The health care sector faces a number of challenges related to the growth of the elderly population, namely, multimodal geriatric syndromes, interdisciplinary care modeling, and understanding the social determinants of illness to develop approaches

---

Box 1
Three principles of action to achieve health equity

1. Improve the conditions of daily life—the circumstances in which people are born, grow, live, work, and age.

2. Tackle the inequitable distribution of power, money, and resources—the structural drivers of those conditions of daily life—globally, nationally, and locally.

3. Measure the problem, evaluate action, expand the knowledge base, develop a workforce that is trained in the social determinants of health, and raise public awareness about the social determinants of health.

From Commission on Social Determinants of Health (CSDH). A new global agenda. In: Closing the gap in a generation: health equity through action on the social determinants of health. Geneva (Switzerland): World Health Organization; 2008. p. 34; with permission.

to minimize the effects. All of these initiatives require a dedicated workforce of professionals to address these issues, which leads to the final trend: availability of the workforce and expanded use of advanced practice nurses.

PROVIDER AVAILABILITY

Dr Pillemer, Chair of the Behavioral and Social Sciences Section, is a Professor in the Department of Human Development, a Professor of Gerontology in Medicine at Weill Cornell Medicine, and the Senior Associate Dean for Research and Outreach in the College of Human Ecology. Dr Pillemer discussed his concern with the shortage of a professional workforce to care for the aging population, especially in conjunction with the explosion of Alzheimer's disease.[11] The need for more health care professionals was also shared by Dr Griebling as one of his major areas of concern for the future.[11]

The redistribution of the population discussed elsewhere in this article will result in a decrease in the relative size of the working population as compared with the nonworking population, along with adding to the need for workers to provide care to the aging population. Cohen[30] shared that there will be a "critical shortage of basic healthcare providers" in the future unless changes are made to the health care labor market.

The World Health Organization took a closer look at this issue in the report, *Global Strategy on Human Resources for Health: Workforce 2030.*[31] Findings from this report identified the supply of health care workers in many countries is insufficient.[31] Estimates could be calculated for only 165 countries owing to lack of available data to model the projections.[31] Projections by 2030 estimate a global deficit of health workers to meet needs at 18 million as compared with 7 million in 2013.[31] The worldwide demand will grow from 48 million in 2013 to more than 80 million in 2030.[31] There is the potential for the creation of nearly 40 million new health care–related jobs using the sample of 165 countries.[31] An additional challenge in the creation of these new jobs is to align the positions in the regions and countries with unmet population needs. The current pace of production will need to be accelerated, as the authors warn against complacency and that maintaining the status quo will result in too slow of progress.[31]

Taking a closer look at nursing, specifically in the United States, Zhang and colleagues[32] updated their prior study on nursing shortages and found 37 of the 50 states will experience significant shortages of nurses by 2030. The Western and Southern regions will experience the greatest shortage, which correlates with the growing elderly populations in these regions.[32] The projected shortfall of 1 million registered nurses in the original report was decreases to 500,000 by 2030.[32] In the area of primary care, it is estimated by 2025 there will be a shortage of nearly 24,000 full-time primary care physicians.[33] Additionally, there is a significant need for geriatricians, as noted by a decrease in geriatric fellows by 22%.[30] Nurse practitioners are predicted to have a surplus in all states and physician assistants will have an anticipated surplus in most states by 2025.[33] Taking a closer look at the trends in primary care delivery between physicians, nurse practitioners, and physician assistants, Xue and colleagues[33] examined a sample of elderly Medicare beneficiaries (2008–2014). Three models were compared: a physician model (MD only), a shared care model (MD and either nurse practitioner or physician assistant), and a nurse practitioner/physician assistant model (either nurse practitioner/physician assistant or both).[33] The physician model remains the most common model, but there was a shift to a greater use of the shared model (from 12% to 23%), whereas the nurse practitioner/physician assistant showed minimal change (from 2.7% to 5.9%).[33] With the effective use of nurse practitioner and physician assistant roles, the shortage of physicians can be mitigated.[33] Xue and colleagues[33] described access to care for the vulnerable elderly population as a national priority and the shift in the shared care model, along with the nurse practitioner/physician assistant model, will work to serve the growing chronic disease burden in the elderly population. Although these are positive trends, there remains significant need for concern and continued proactive strategies.

The shortage of health care workers is a critical issue facing the health care delivery system not only in the United States, but globally. High-quality care cannot be attained without a system that supplies adequately trained providers. The financing to support a system that prioritizes quality and health is essential for success because the economy will be strained with the increased demand of resources brought on by the growing elderly population.

FINANCIAL IMPACT OF HEALTH

Each of the panelists touched on some aspect of financing during the webinar or within their respective trend report. The vast range of issues (reimbursement, the Affordable Care Act, federal research funding, and Supplemental Securities Income) mentioned were broad and cannot be fully addressed in this article.[3–6,11] Instead, an overview of changes in reimbursement and the importance of investing in health from a broad view will be addressed.

The Quality Payment Program was established by the Medicare Access and CHIP Reauthorization Act of 2015 as a quality incentive program for qualifying physicians and advanced practice nurses.[34] Reimbursement is based on value over volume referred to as the Merit-Based Incentive Payment System. The shift is to move from a fee-for-service model to linking payment to outcomes and quality. The system is currently in the second year of implementation (2018), with initial data collection on the performance measures collected in 2017.[34] The first payment adjustment will be made beginning January 2019 for those who qualify.[34] Merit-Based Incentive Payment System performance categories for 2018 include quality (50%), cost (10%), improvement activities (15%), and advancing care information (25%).[34] A total Merit-Based Incentive Payment System score will be calculated to determine payment, which will range from ±4% in 2019 and adjust up to ±9% in 2022.[34] In the area of quality, the practitioner chooses 6 items out of the list of quality measures (217 measures available for 2018) for reporting.[34] As an example, patient frailty evaluation is included on the list of quality measures. Cost will be calculated for Medicare spending per beneficiary and total per capita costs.[34] Improvement activities offers a list of 113 options for the practitioner to choose from, including improve health status of the community, improve self-care, and chronic disease prevention and self-management program.[34] Advancing care information centers on interoperability. In 2018, there is a bonus point structure available for treating complex patients with applicable performance submission.[34] The system change was designed to meet the Centers for Medicare and Medicaid Services overarching goals of better care, smarter spending, and healthier people.[34]

The importance of focusing on health not only from the perspective of improving or extending people's lives, but it also has an overall economic benefit. In low- and middle-income countries, health improvement has accounted for approximately an 11% economic growth.[35] This number is as high as 24%, when the value of additional lives (VLYs) was included.[35] VLYs is the intrinsic value of benefit of health that leads to a higher life expectancy (decrease mortality)—the authors refer to VLYs and economic growth as full income.[35] Full income provides a more complete view of health's contribution to the well-being of a country.[35] The authors propose that, by including VLYs in projections for economic benefits, a greater proportion of assistance could be allocated for health because it would reflect a stronger return on investment.[35] Jamison and colleagues[35] shared by using VLYs between 2015 and 2035 the estimate of economic benefit would exceed costs by a factor of 9 to 20, supporting a very attractive investment argument. Understanding the value of health improvement from an economic standpoint provides a strong rationale for improved resource allocation to health and health-related resources.

To gain financial support for research, new programs, education, recruitment, certifications, and other initiatives to address the issues related to the growing aging population, an argument must be made to elicit the interest of policymakers and decision makers. The financial value to a country by reducing mortality while achieving a substantial return on investment, in the face of a surge in elderly population, provides support for further discussion to direct investment in health care programs to address these pertinent issues.

SUMMARY

The increased life expectancy and volume of the older population will have a significant impact on health care services in the future. Providers are challenged to examine the current health care structure and evaluate changes in approaches to align with the change in the population landscape. The historical approach of traditional medicine and models of care based on standalone and acute care treatments will no longer be effective with the more complex, multifaceted issues involving older individuals with multiple chronic conditions. This changing environment requires a different perspective that includes seeking collaboration across disciplines with the goal of simultaneous and coordinated interventions. Interprofessional syndrome care is needed to avoid negative interactions among treatment plans for different conditions, such as polypharmacy.

Social and health determinants of care are essential to incorporate in treatment planning because these factors are linked to higher rates of geriatric syndromes. Conditions such as frailty and other geriatric syndromes require a concerted effort to incorporate screening, assessment, and individualized care planning to address quality of life and reduce mortality risk. The complex conditions facing the growing geriatric population will require innovative approaches.

Advanced practice nurses are positioned to positively effect changes in the care of the geriatric population. The increasing availability of advanced practice nurses aligning with the significant need for primary care providers provides an opportunity to develop expertise in geriatric care. Every setting will be challenged with designing effective, quality-driven delivery systems. Advanced practice nurses can be at the forefront of every aspect of geriatric care, from piloting multidisciplinary care models to being a voice for change in sharing the impact of patient experiences as it relates to seeking health equity.

The Centers for Medicare and Medicaid Services has outlined in the revised payment model the support for change. The plan to drive greater collaborative practice and open avenues for advanced practice nurses to establish practice models to achieve improved care are essential to stimulate needed change. Designing the program with quality outcomes as the means for payment adjustments clearly outlines a priority shift from volume to value.

The GSA, through the trend reports and subsequent webinar, provided the foundation for this article to stimulate continued discussion and exploration of key factors facing the care of the elderly.[3–6,11] Widening our knowledge and perspective of the aging population across disciplines and focus areas can lead to a more prepared workforce in planning for the future.

REFERENCES

1. (GSA) GS of A. Purpose and mission. Available at: https://www.geron.org/about-us/purposes-and-mission. Accessed November 1, 2018.
2. Posey LM. 2018 trends in the health sciences 2018. Available at: https://www.geron.org/images/membership/HealthSciencesTrendsReport2018.pdf. Accessed October 30, 2018.
3. Posey LM. Trends in social research, policy, and practice 2017. Available at: https://www.geron.org/images/membership/SRPPTrends2017.pdf. Accessed November 1, 2018.
4. Posey LM. Trends in the behavioral and social sciences 2017. Available at: https://www.geron.org/images/membership/2017_GSA_TrendsinAging_BSS_Final.pdf. Accessed October 30, 2018.
5. Nikolich-Zugich J. Trends in the biological sciences 2016. Washington, DC.
6. Griebling TL. Trends in the health sciences 2017. Available at: https://www.geron.org/images/membership/2017HSTrendsReport.pdf. Accessed October 30, 2018.
7. Posey LM. 2018 trends in social research, policy, and practice 2018. Available at: https://www.geron.org/images/membership/SRPPTrends2018.pdf. Accessed November 1, 2018.
8. Ortman JM, Velkoff VA, Hogan H. An aging nation: the older population in the United States. population estimates and projections. Curr Popul Rep 2014;1964. https://doi.org/10.1016/j.jaging.2004.02.002.
9. Roberts AW, Ogunwole SU, Blakeslee L, et al. The population 65 years and older in the United States: 2016 American Community survey reports 2018. Available at: www.census.gov/acs. Accessed October 30, 2018.
10. Association AP. Aging and socioeconomic status 2018. Available at: https://www.apa.org/pi/ses/resources/publications/age.aspx. Accessed October 30, 2018.
11. (GSA) GS of A. GSA need to know webinar series 2017 trends in aging. Available at: https://www.youtube.com/watch?v=JkG3BWKNqww&feature=youtu.be. Accessed November 1, 2018.
12. Palmer K, Onder G, Cesari M. The geriatric condition of frailty. Eur J Intern Med 2018;56:1–2.
13. de Llano PM, Lange C, Nunes DP, et al. Frailty in rural older adults: development of a care algorithm. Acta Paul Enferm 2017;30(5):520–30.
14. Sloane PD, Cesari M. Research on frailty: continued progress, continued challenges. J Am Med Dir Assoc 2018;19(4):279–81.
15. World Health Organization (WHO). Reprinted from: world report on ageing and health: chapter 3: health in older age 2015. Available at: http://www.who.int/ageing/publications/world-report-2015/en/. Accessed November 10, 2018.
16. Chen X, Mao G, Leng SX. Frailty syndrome: an overview. Clin Interv Aging 2014;9:433–41.
17. Calvani R, Marini F, Cesari M, et al. Biomarkers for physical frailty and sarcopenia. Aging Clin Exp Res 2017;29(1):29–34.
18. Theou O, Squires E, Mallery K, et al. What do we know about frailty in the acute care setting? A scoping review. BMC Geriatr 2018;18(1). https://doi.org/10.1186/s12877-018-0823-2.

19. Inzitari M, Pérez LM, Enfedaque MB, et al. Integrated primary and geriatric care for frail older adults in the community: implementation of a complex intervention into real life. Eur J Intern Med 2018;56:57–63.

20. Chen CY, Gan P, How CH. Approach to frailty in the elderly in primary care and the community. Singapore Med J 2018;59(5):240–5.

21. Searle SD, Rockwood K. What proportion of older adults in hospital are frail? Lancet 2018;391(10132):1751–2.

22. Cesari M, Marzetti E, Thiem U, et al. The geriatric management of frailty as paradigm of the end of the disease era. Eur J Intern Med 2016;31(2016):11–4.

23. Hansen KT, McDonald C, O'Hara S, et al. A formative evaluation of a nurse practitioner-led interprofessional geriatric outpatient clinic. J Interprof Care 2017;31(4):546–9.

24. Mudge AM, Banks MD, Barnett AG, et al. CHERISH (collaboration for hospitalised elders reducing the impact of stays in hospital): protocol for a multi-site improvement program to reduce geriatric syndromes in older inpatients. BMC Geriatr 2017;17(1):1–9.

25. de Vos A, Cramm JM, van Wijngaarden JDH, et al. Understanding implementation of comprehensive geriatric care programs: a multiple perspective approach is preferred. Int J Health Plann Manage 2017;32(4):608–36.

26. LaVeist T, Gaskin D, Richard P. The economic burden of health inequalities in the United States 2009. Washington, DC.

27. World Health Organization. Final Report on the Commission on Social Determinants of Health. Geneva (Switzerland): Commission on Social Determinants of Health (CSDH); 2008.

28. Reutter L, Kushner K. Health equity through action on the social determinants of health. Nurs Inq 2008;17(3):269–80.

29. (CSDH) C on SD of H. Reprinted from: closing the gap in a generation: health equity through action on the social determinants of health: chapter 16: the social determinants of health: monitoring, research and training 2008. Available at: http://www.who.int/social_determinants/thecommission/finalreport/en/.

30. Cohen S. A review of demographic and infrastructural factors and potential solutions to the physician and nursing shortage predicted to impact the growing US elderly population. J Public Health Manag Pract 2009;15(4):352–62.

31. World Health Organization (WHO). Reprinted from: global strategy on human resources for health: Geneva (Switzerland): Workforce 2030 2016. https://doi.org/10.1017/CBO9781107415324.004. Annex 1. Accessed November 10, 2018.

32. Zhang X, Tai D, Pforsich H, et al. United States registered nurse workforce report card and shortage forecast: a revisit. Am J Med Qual 2018;33(3):229–36.

33. Xue Y, Goodwin JS, Adhikari D, et al. Trends in primary care provision to Medicare beneficiaries by physicians, nurse practitioners, or physician assistants: 2008-2014. J Prim Care Community Health 2017;8(4):256–63.

34. Chalick-Kaplan B, Conners B. MIPS: what you need to know in year 2- A conversation with CMS. Philadelphia: CMS; 2017. Available at: https://vimeo.com/247223899.

35. Jamison DT, Summers LH, Alleyne G, et al. Global health 2035: a world converging within a generation. Lancet 2013;383(9908):1898–955.

Treatment and Outcomes in Adult Designated Psychiatric Emergency Service Units

Linda Ledet, DNS, APRN, PMHCNS-BC[a],*,
Benita N. Chatmon, PhD, MSN, RN, CNE[b]

KEYWORDS

- Emergency care • Mental health • Designated care • Behavioral health
- Psychiatric emergency services

KEY POINTS

- There are many challenges in caring for the psychiatric patient in a crisis.
- Traditional emergency service departments increase stress on psychiatric patients and hospital staff.
- Designated psychiatric emergency service units enhance patient care by providing for rapid assessment, safe environments, enhanced specialized care, and appropriate disposition on discharge.
- Experienced psychiatric clinicians can positively affect outcomes of psychiatric patients in designated psychiatric emergency service emergency departments with specialized emergency care.

INTRODUCTION

Mental health emergency department (ED) visits are increasing steadily. It is estimated that 6% to 9% of all ED visits are related to patients with a mental disorder.[1] EDs had a 4-fold increase in the ratio of patients presenting with mental illness compared with other types of health problems in the last decade.[2] These numbers reflect the crisis in our mental health system. Overuse of the ED by mental health patients and the ongoing problem of poor access to appropriate psychiatric care affect emergency

Disclosure Statement: The authors do not have any relationships with a commercial company that has a direct financial interest in the subject matter or materials discussed in article or with a company making a competing product.
[a] School of Nursing, LSU Health New Orleans, 1900 Gravier Street, Office 4A13, New Orleans, LA 70112, USA; [b] School of Nursing, LSU Health New Orleans, 1900 Gravier Street, Office 331, New Orleans, LA 70112, USA
* Corresponding author.
E-mail address: llede3@lsuhsc.edu

Crit Care Nurs Clin N Am 31 (2019) 225–236
https://doi.org/10.1016/j.cnc.2019.02.008
0899-5885/19/© 2019 Elsevier Inc. All rights reserved.

services.[3] Overuse and overcrowding in EDs may limit the availability of ED staff, ED beds for other patients, and longer wait times for all patients.[4] Safety is of primary concern when having mental health patients in general EDs due to environmental hazards and inappropriate care.

Often individuals with mental illness wait too long to seek care, resulting in a mental health crisis. This crisis results in patients using EDs as a treatment option. Mental health patients in the ED board for long hours to days waiting for available transfer to appropriate inpatient psychiatric beds. Boarding is a costly practice for both the patient and the hospital because the mentally ill patient is not receiving the appropriate care that they need, and the hospital is incurring financial expenses and staff stress. Negative experiences and outcomes are frequently reported in general EDs by patients in a mental health crisis, such as an escalation of psychiatric symptoms, safety issues for patients and staff, patient boarding, high cost, and delayed time to triage and discharge.[3,4]

Patients experiencing a mental health crisis deserve to be cared for in a safe environment that is suitable for appropriate assessment and care. Often, general EDs are noisy environments that are unsafe for a person in a mental health crisis. Meeting the needs of mentally ill patients in a general ED is a challenge. It is imperative that psychiatric patients in crisis receive prompt attention in a safe environment. Psychiatric cases that present in general EDs may not receive specialized psychiatric care from health care workers trained in mental health in a timely fashion.[4] According to the Joint Commission, creating a designated psychiatric emergency service (PES) unit can assist hospitals in alleviating boarding of psychiatric patients.[5] In the last decade, emergency care for patients with mental health needs is moving toward designated PES units with specialized care for the patient with mental health needs. A designated PES unit is a stand-alone ED providing specialized psychiatric care and is usually affiliated with an adjacent medical ED.[6] General or medical EDs provide care for all types of patients in crisis and do not specialize in care for the mentally ill. The aim of this article is to discuss treatment and outcomes of adult psychiatric patients in designated PES units.

TRIAGE OF THE PSYCHIATRIC PATIENT

Triage is the process whereby patients presenting into the emergency room are rated based on their clinical urgency.[7–9] Triage is typically associated with urgent physical issues and was not suited ideally for psychosocial issues until recent years.[9,10] There is a clear difference between medical and psychiatric emergencies when triaging a patient. The medical triage process involves urgent evaluations and prioritization of patients' medical disposition following a medical assessment. The triage process is based on a threat to life or complication of a disease process. In contrast, psychiatric emergencies involve triage of the level of danger the patient presents to others and themselves. Triage also involves the severity of their social functioning. Hence, specific tools to triage psychiatric patients are vital when trying to improve nursing assessment of patients with mental health problems, improve the triage process, reduce wait time, and manage resources.[9]

Several mental health triage tools exist that could be initiated in PES units across the United States. The Australian Mental Health Triage Scale, Risk Assessment Matrix, and Canadian Triage and Acuity Scale are some triage scales specific to the psychiatric patient.[9,11,12] This article specifically addresses the Australian Mental Health Triage Scale (formerly known as the Mental Health Triage Scale) due to its ability to produce shorter wait times, improve nurses' confidence in triaging patient with mental health presentations, as well as reduce the time to intervention and assessment. Furthermore, the Australian Mental Health Triage Scale has been extensively researched as a comprehensive and effective tool for the assessment of mental illness presentation.[9,10]

Smart and colleagues[9] developed the Australian Mental Health Triage Scale, which merged psychiatric patients into the National Triage Scale. This integration was done to improve nurses' assessments of patients with mental health issues, improve the effectiveness of the triage of mental health presentation, and decrease the time from triage to medical assessment, as well as the time from triage until discharge from the ED. The Australian Mental Health Triage Scale prioritizes patients based on behavioral presentation while placing time parameters on the evaluation of the psychiatric patient. The Australian Mental Health Triage Scale consist of five categories:

Category 1	Immediately life threatening, severe behavioral disturbances, patient must be seen immediately
Category 2	Emergency: patient is violent, aggressive, or suicidal and must be seen within 10 min
Category 3	Urgent: patient is very distressed or acutely psychotic and must be seen within 30 min
Category 4	Semi-urgent: patient has a well-established psychiatric disorder and must be seen within 60 min
Category 5	Nonurgent: patient has a well-established, nonacute psychiatric disorder and should be seen within 120 min

Following the development and initiation of the Australian Mental Health Triage Scale, the mean waiting times reduced from 34.3 minutes to 29.1 minutes and the mean time to disposition reduced from 149.2 minutes to 131.8 minutes. As a result, a reduction of 88.9 patient hours occurred over a 3-month period.[9,10]

SIGNIFICANCE OF THE PROBLEM

Evaluation of the psychiatric patient can take place in psychiatric inpatient and outpatient settings, as well as general medical settings. The latter setting, however, creates obstacles when attempting to observe risky behaviors and provide interventions for the psychiatric patient. To begin with, the staff on a general medical setting are not trained to assess psychiatric patients, hence their observational skills tend to be less than those of staff trained on a psychiatric unit.[13] Lack of key observational skills for the psychiatric patient population can serve as a safety hazard. Further, there are constant interruptions and lack of privacy in general medical settings, which can prohibit the clinician from obtaining key assessment details.[13] Similarly, the general ED provides a broad spectrum of care to emergent and/or critical care conditions. The broad spectrum of the ED results in a care environment that is not conducive to taking care of the psychiatric population.[14]

There are approximately 12 million psychiatric visits to hospital EDs a year.[15] In addition, psychiatric patients are more likely to revisit EDs than patients without psychiatric conditions.[14,15] Various factors contribute to readmission of psychiatric patients. These factors include unavailability of outpatient providers, lack of ability of the patient to cope with their mental health condition, and treatment noncompliance.[14] The frequent readmissions as well as lack of placement have led to patient boarding becoming a major problem across EDs in the United States.[1,16]

Boarding occurs when patients, in particular psychiatric patients, have to withstand long holding periods until a psychiatric inpatient bed is available. This wait could range anywhere from 6.8 hours to 34 hours.[1] Some reasons for boarding psychiatric patients include:

1. Decreased availability of psychiatric clinicians to evaluate the patient
2. Absence of resources to conduct psychiatric evaluations such as mental health assessment tools
3. Insufficient number of lower levels of outpatient care and services
4. Requirements for pre-authorization of insurance before admission[1]

These long boarding times are challenging to health care facilities from both a financial and medical standpoint. Boarding of patients cost a health care facilities' ED approximately $2264 per stay. During the boarding period, patients can become hostile and their symptoms may become progressively worst. Many facilities board their psychiatric patients in EDs either with a police officer or near the nursing station; given the safety risk with this type of placement, consideration of the environment is imperative with regard to not only staff but also other patients.[10] Appropriate evaluation of psychiatric patients can occur when these patients transfer from a general ED to a psychiatric ED.[1,16] The significance of having dedicated PES units includes mobilizing effective standards of care, reduction of wait time, and an alternative to boarding for the psychiatric patient.[1]

FOCUSED MEDICAL ASSESSMENT/CLEARANCE

A focused medical assessment is conducted to evaluate a patient for the existence of an emergency medical condition that would warrant treatment. During the medical assessment, the clinician first obtains a history and a physical examination. If the client is having an acute psychotic episode, stabilization of client signs and symptoms may have to take precedence over the history and physical examination. The clinician may need to elicit answers from family and friends of the patient to complete the patient's history. Next, the clinician needs to assess if the patient is intoxicated or under the influence of illegal or legal drugs. Furthermore, the clinician then assesses if the patient's symptoms are being exacerbated by a medical condition and if they are, treat and/or stabilize the medical condition. After completion of laboratory or radiologic tests and the medical assessment, if the clinician finds no known medical cause, the patient is noted to be medically stable and may then undergo psychiatric evaluation.[10]

Slade and colleagues[10] reported that medical clearance should demonstrate that without a reasonable doubt, there are no contributory factors to the patient's presenting psychiatric complaints, no medical emergency, and the patient is medically stable to be transferred to the intended or appropriate clinical services. All health care agencies were encouraged to establish recommendations for psychiatric patients with low medical risk.[10] **Box 1** contains an example of criteria for low medical risk.

Box 1
Criteria for psychiatric patients with low medical risk

Age between 15 and 55 years

No acute medical complaints

No evidence of a pattern of substance abuse (alcohol or drug)

Normal physical examination

Data from Slade M, Taber D, Clarke M, et al. Best practices for the treatment of patients with mental and substance use illnesses in the emergency department. Dis Mon 2007;53(11–12):536–80.

These criteria considered age, medical complaint, history of substance abuse, and a normal physical examination. A normal physical examination consisted of normal vital signs, gait, strength, fluency of speech, memory, and concentration. Despite medical clearance, patients with chronic medical conditions may require further evaluation at a later time, and patients may have undiagnosed needs that are yet to be discovered.[10]

EMERGENCY PSYCHIATRIC EVALUATION

Psychiatric evaluations usually cannot be fully completed in emergency situations and will vary according to their purpose during crisis. Rapid intervention is based on minimal evidence and data collected in crisis. The provider must attempt to assess the crisis that the patient is experiencing and adjust the psychiatric evaluation process to maintain the safety and stabilization of the patient as quickly as possible. After the patient is stable, the process of a full psychiatric evaluation is then possible. Definitive diagnosis is not considered a primary goal of the initial ED assessment, however investigation as to whether the patient has an underlying medical problem should be addressed early in the assessment and medical clearance.[17] Developing a provisional, differential diagnosis based on assessment findings and identifying causes or contributing factors to the patient's emergent situation aim to guide the appropriate plan of care.[17]

Emergency care in PES units includes visual observation of the patient's behavior and verbal and nonverbal interactions, before direct patient interview. The primary source for data collection and assessment is the patient; however, often the patient is not a reliable source of information and history. Multiple sources of secondary information may be obtained from individuals who accompany the patient, such as family, friends, emergency personnel, and/or police officers.[17] Medical records of the patient may be useful to determine previous medications, diagnosis, and treatments. Relevant information can be shared with those professionals collaborating directly in the patient's care.[18]

The patient's chief complaint and reason for coming to the PES unit must be elicited. The clinician should develop a therapeutic relationship with the patient so that trust can encourage information sharing. To facilitate a therapeutic relationship, it is important to demonstrate empathy toward the patient's distress and complaints. The patient's vital signs are taken during triage if possible. A brief history, including the present and past psychiatric and medical history, are obtained. Also, the nurse explores substance use, social history, and family history. Initial assessment and mental status examination may be challenging but should occur during the interview process. The mental status examination includes appearance, attitude, behavior, mood and affect, thought content/processes, perceptions, cognition, insight, and judgment. If the patient is agitated, de-escalation is essential for the safety of the patient and others in the environment. The assessment and interview may have to wait until the patient has calmed down. Verbal communication, de-escalation techniques, and pharmacologic management may be useful in calming the patient down. Restraints and seclusion are considered a last resort intervention only after all other de-escalation techniques are attempted and physical danger is an immediate concern.

Safety Assessment

During the initial assessment, the immediate concern is to assess and enhance the safety of the patient and others. Suicidal ideation is often a presenting psychiatric complaint in the ED. The literature acknowledges several suicide risk assessment tools, but none were found to be helpful predictors.[19] Risk factors for suicide that have been identified are male gender, age (less than 19 years and over 45 years), ethnicity of white or native American, unmarried, gay or lesbian youth, previous suicide attempt, presence of a psychiatric diagnosis, guilt, states desire to die, substance abuse, previous inpatient admission, depression, anxiety, lack of social support, living alone, recent loss, chronic pain and/or debilitating physical illness, and access to means to inflict harm.[19] Protective factors include the ability to identify reasons for living, responsibility for the care of others, having custodial children, strong spiritual beliefs against violence and suicide, and engagement in school and work.[17] Clinicians should ask specific questions related to suicidal and homicidal thoughts and behaviors to determine the nature of thoughts, plan details, and means to carry out the plan. Homicidal patients undergo a similar risk assessment, which includes history, collateral information, desire to harm others with a plan, and means to carry out the plan.[16] A search of the patient and their belongings for weapons or potential weapons during initial assessment is warranted. The process of suicide assessment is based on clinical judgment related to available information and behaviors to determine the likelihood of suicide or harm.[17] Designated PES units can provide ideal environments to keep a patient safe and continuously monitored on suicide precautions until further disposition is determined. Designated PES units are designed to be environmentally safe spaces to treat patients with safety concerns.

Cognitive Assessment

The patient's cognitive status is part of the initial psychiatric evaluation. Presentation of cognitive impairment because of delirium is a medical emergency. Delirium is a serious mental disturbance that occurs usually rapidly over hours to days. Delirium presents with confused thinking and reduced awareness and/or inattention. In the medical assessment and clearance, it is essential to discover and treat the contributing factor of the delirium rapidly, because the prognosis greatly decreases within days of development of the state of delirium. A history from caregivers, friends, and/or family members is essential, because the cognitively impaired patient may be unable to fully participate in the psychiatric interview process. The Folstein Mini Mental State Examination (MMSE) is a useful cognitive screening instrument.[20] The MMSE is a structured 30-point questionnaire used extensively in clinical settings.

Intoxication/Withdrawal Assessment

Clinicians in PES units should observe and evaluate the patient for signs of intoxication or withdrawal. Intoxicated patients should receive care in a regular ED and be monitored closely until they are sober and are safe to treat in the designated PES unit. Psychiatric patients who present with signs and symptoms of acute psychosis, severe anxiety or agitation, mania, and present a safety risk, such as gravely disabled, require psychiatric evaluation in the designated PES unit. A Physicians Emergency Certificate is executed before or in the PES unit when an individual is a danger to self, others, and/or gravely disabled. As a result of a mental disorder, a gravely disabled person is in serious danger because they are unable to provide for their essential human health and/or safety needs. It is helpful to obtain a history from the patient if possible and supplement with information from family or significant others in emergencies.

MEDICATION

The American College of Emergency Physicians made a few recommendations for patients who may or may not have a psychiatric experience.[10] They recommend the use of benzodiazepines and antipsychotic medications for those patients experiencing agitation and are cooperative.[10] **Table 1** describes the medication recommendations for patients in designated PES units.

The appropriate management of an agitated patient is essential to the safety of staff and other patients, as well as the suitability of the treatment plan for the patient. In most situations, nonpharmacologic interventions are the first-line approach for patients in acute settings. Nonpharmacologic interventions include behavioral controls or even nicotine replacement therapy. Furthermore, pharmacologic approaches are considered when symptoms are extreme or disabling and when a risk of notable harm exists. The goal of medication administration is to calm the patient so that the clinician can appropriately and accurately assess the patient.

Three medication classes most often used in treating agitations include first-generation (typical) antipsychotics (FGAs), second-generation (atypical) antipsychotics (SGAs), and benzodiazepines.[21] Evidence has shown that typical antipsychotics, atypical antipsychotics, and benzodiazepines, whether used alone or in combination, are effective agents for calming patients rapidly.[21,22] Lorazepam (Ativan) is the benzodiazepine of choice for acute management of violent behavior. However, second-generation antipsychotic medications such as olanzapine (Zyprexa) and ziprasidone (Geodan) are commonly used due to their reduced side effects compared with FGAs. However, directly addressing the underlying cause of the agitation is the definitive and preferred treatment of choice for patients experiencing acute anxiety and agitation.

FIRST-GENERATION ANTIPSYCHOTICS

First-generation antipsychotics have a lengthy history of use for agitation. First-generation antipsychotics inhibit dopamine transmission in the human brain, which most likely causes a calming effect. Chlorpromazine (Thorazine) was the first FGA approved and marketed by the U.S. Food and Drug Administration. Chlorpromazine has a tendency to cause more hypotension, lower seizure threshold, and has more anticholinergic side effects than haloperidol (Haldol). Hence, chlorpromazine is not recommended for use in acute agitation. FGA medications, such as haloperidol, historically have been the mostly widely used medication for aggressive and violent patients. Haloperidol has few effects on vital signs, anticholinergic activity, and minimum interaction with other antipsychiatric medications. The most taxing consequences of haloperidol are the extrapyramidal symptoms. Extrapyramidal symptoms affect limbic

Table 1
Recommendations for medication use for patients in designated psychiatric emergency services

Patient Presentation	Cooperation	Medication Recommendation
Acutely agitated (nonpsychotic)	Cooperative	Oral benzodiazepine
Acutely agitated (nonpsychotic)	Uncooperative	IM benzodiazepine
Acutely agitated (psychotic)	Cooperative	Dissolving oral antipsychotic
Acutely agitated (psychotic)	Uncooperative	Injection of antipsychotic
Psychiatric history without agitation with symptoms such as irritability or anxiety	Cooperative/ uncooperative	Benzodiazepine for anxiety Antipsychotic for psychotic symptoms

Data from Slade M, Taber D, Clarke M, et al. Best practices for the treatment of patients with mental and substance use illnesses in the emergency department. Dis Mon 2007;53(11–12):536–80.

and motor centers. Patients experiencing extrapyramidal symptoms may experience acute dystonia, akathisia, and pseudoparkinsonism symptoms.[21]

SECOND-GENERATION ANTIPSYCHOTICS

Second-generation antipsychotics include serotonin and dopamine antagonists. These medications were mostly developed after the 1990s. Second-generation antipsychotics include clozapine (Clozaril), olanzapine (Zyprexa), risperidone (Risperdal), quetiapine (Seroquel), and ziprasidone (Geodon).[21,23] According to Wilson and colleagues,[23] all of the SGAs are effective in reducing agitation compared with placebo except for risperidone. Clozapine was the first SGA on the market and was shown to dramatically improve symptoms in psychiatric patients who were resistant to FGAs. Moreover, it improved negative symptoms as well.[21] Conversely, clozapine also caused agranulocytosis, myocarditis, and bowel emergencies. Furthermore, SGAs carry the risk of metabolic syndrome, including weight gain, particularly in the abdomen, increased blood glucose levels, insulin resistance, and hyperlipidemia.[21]

BENZODIAZEPINE

According to Slade and colleagues,[10] acutely agitated (nonpsychotic) patients should receive oral benzodiazepines such as lorazepam (Ativan), alprazolam (Xanax), or diazepam (Valium).[21] Benzodiazepines such as lorazepam have been shown to reduce the amount of antipsychotic medications needed for an aggressive or violent patient.[21] Benzodiazepines act on the γ-aminobutyric acid receptor, which is the main inhibitory neurotransmitter in the human brain.[23] All benzodiazepines cause sedation when given in high therapeutic doses. Clinicians prefer benzodiazepines when the patient comes in with ethanol withdrawal, stimulant intoxication, or when the cause of agitation cannot be determined.[23]

Moreover, clinicians prescribe combination drug treatments using antipsychotics and benzodiazepines for patients experiencing agitation. For example, benztropine (Cogentin) use is highly encouraged when haloperidol (Haldol) is given. Benztropine reduces the possibility of extrapyramidal side effects. Similarly, clinicians prescribe perphenazine, lorazepam, and diphenhydramine, or benztropine for some patients experiencing agitation.

Clinicians must assess the appropriateness of the antianxiety and/or antipsychotic medication used in managing aggressive and violent patients. **Table 2** summarizes drugs used to treat acute violent behavior. Long-term treatment of violent and aggressive patients will require treatment of the underlying psychiatric condition.[21]

General recommendations for treatment of agitation include the following:

- Clinicians should avoid using medication as a restraint.
- Nonpharmacologic approaches should be the first treatment approach.
- Medications should be used to calm patients, not to trigger or induce sleep.
- Patient involvement in medication adherence is vital.
- Oral medication is the preferred method of medication administration over the intramuscular route.[23]

OUTCOMES OF A DESIGNATED PSYCHIATRIC EMERGENCY SERVICE UNIT

The prevalent outcome of a designated PES unit is timely stabilization of acute psychiatric crisis while maintaining safety until appropriate patient disposition. Studies

Table 2 Drugs used for acute management of violent behavior			
Antianxiety Agents (Benzodiazepines)	First-Generation Antipsychotics	Second-Generation Antipsychotics	Combinations
Lorazepam (Ativan)	Haloperidol (Haldol)	Risperidone (Risperdal)	Haloperidol (Haldol), lorazepam (Ativan), and diphenhydramine (Benadryl) or benztropine (Cogentin)
Alprazolam (Xanax)	Perphenazine	Olanzapine (Zyprexa, Zydis)	Perphenazine, lorazepam (Ativan), and diphenhydramine (Benadryl), or benztropine (Cogentin)
Diazepam (Valium)	Chlorpromazine (Thorazine) Loxapine (Adasuve)	Ziprasidone (Geodon)	

Data from Farrohknia N, Castrén M, Ehrenberg A, et al. Emergency department triage scales and their components: a systematic review of the scientific evidence. Scand J Trauma Resusc Emerg Med 2011;19(1):42.

demonstrate that designated PES units improve timely access to care and cost savings from reduced boarding times for patients awaiting psychiatric care.[1,17] The maximum PES visit of 20 hours at $110 per hour costs less overall than the current estimate of $2264 for an average ED boarding and the thousands of dollars saved by avoiding a psychiatric hospitalization.[1,24] Comparing the cost of the maximum PES unit visit with the average ED boarding may not seem significant, however considering that psychiatric symptoms often escalate while boarding in the ED, that in turn may lead to costly psychiatric hospitalization.[24] Designated PES units reduced the length of boarding times for patients awaiting psychiatric care by over 80% versus comparable state ED averages.[1] Such outcomes are aligned with health care reform of improving access to care and lowering health care cost.

Other positive patient outcomes are reduced waiting times and reduced use of restraints.[1,15] A designated PES unit provides a comfortable and calm environment for the patient, because they are assessed and evaluated in a less restrictive care option for crisis stabilization.[25] A designated PES unit can dramatically alleviate the demand of inpatient psychiatric beds compared with a general ED by providing immediate assessment and treatment.[25] Designated PES units provide assessment and treatment in patients experiencing a mental health crisis, thus alleviating the need for inpatient disposition in 75% of patients.[1] Most psychiatric crises can be stabilized in less than 24 hours in a PES unit with appropriate interventions, thus averting the need for inpatient hospitalization.[1] In a study conducted in the Sacramento region, improved and timely access to care, decreased boarding times, and decreased hospitalization cost identified the designated PES unit as a worthy part of the mental health care delivery system.[25] The literature has identified several benefits to PES units (**Box 2**). There is a paucity of research investigating the outcomes of designated PES units, however all of the studies reviewed reported favorable outcomes. More research is needed regarding designated PES units for evidence-based practice.

Box 2
Benefits of PES units

Decreased boarding times

ED cost savings

Reduced wait times

Timely stabilization of patient

Prevention of self-harm

Prevention of harm to others

Reduced use of physical restraints

Enhance mental health patient care

Decreased staff stress in medical ED

Patient satisfaction

Connection to appropriate resources/referrals

SUMMARY

The national trend of decreasing the number of state psychiatric beds and resources continues to have devastating effects on the treatment of acutely and chronically ill psychiatric patients. As a result, the numbers of psychiatric patients using general EDs have continued to increase, resulting in a magnitude of issues, such as overcrowding, boarding, unsafe environments for patients, staff stress, and excessive cost. Psychiatric patients in crisis need timely, appropriate, and safe care. Caring for patients in a psychiatric crisis in a general ED can be challenging and lead to stress for both the patient and the staff. A designated PES ED can provide psychiatric patients with specialized emergency care to improve treatment outcomes, decrease unproductive boarding practices, and develop the most appropriate disposition plans with the information gathered during the assessment/evaluation process. The safety and stabilization of the patient are crucial components in the process of caring for the psychiatric patient in crisis. A designated PES unit, within or adjacent to an ED, is equipped to provide for the needs of a psychiatric patient in crisis while maximizing the appropriate resources and outcomes.

REFERENCES

1. Zeller S, Calma N, Stone A. Effect of a regional dedicated psychiatric emergency service on boarding and hospitalization of psychiatric patients in area Emergency Departments. West J Emerg Med 2014;15(1):1–6.

2. Brennaman L. Exceeding the legal time limits for involuntary mental health examinations. Policy Polit Nurs Pract 2015;16(3–4):67–78.

3. Alakeson V, Pande N, Ludwig M. A plan to reduce emergency room 'boarding' of psychiatric patients. Health Aff 2010;29(9):1637–42.

4. Falvo T, Grove L, Stachura R, et al. The opportunity loss of boarding admitted patients in the Emergency Department. Acad Emerg Med 2007;14(4):332–7. https://doi.org/10.1197/j.aem.2006.11.011.

5. The Joint Commission. Alleviating ED boarding of psychiatric patients. Quick Safety 2015;(19):1–3. Available at: https://www.jointcommission.org/assets/1/23/Quick_Safety_Issue_19_Dec_20151.pdf. Accessed December 11, 2018.
6. Zeller S. Treatment of psychiatric patents in emergency settings. Prim Psychiatry 2010;17(6):41–7.
7. Clarke D, Boyce-Gaudreau K, Sanderson A, et al. ED triage decision-making with mental health presentations: a "think aloud" study. J Emerg Nurs 2015;41(6):496–502.
8. Farrohknia N, Castrén M, Ehrenberg A, et al. Emergency Department triage scales and their components: a systematic review of the scientific evidence. Scand J Trauma Resusc Emerg Med 2011;19(1):42.
9. Smart D, Pollard C, Walpole B. Mental health triage in emergency medicine. Aust N Z J Psychiatry 1999;33:57–66.
10. Slade M, Taber D, Clarke M, et al. Best practices for the treatment of patients with mental and substance use illnesses in the Emergency Department. Dis Mon 2007;53(11–12):536–80.
11. Molina-López A, Cruz-Islas J, Palma-Cortés M, et al. Validity and reliability of a novel Color-Risk Psychiatric Triage in a psychiatric emergency department. BMC Psychiatry 2016;16(1). https://doi.org/10.1186/s12888-016-0727-7.
12. Patel A, Harrison A, Bruce-Jones W. Evaluation of the risk assessment matrix: a mental health triage tool. Emerg Med J 2009;26(1):11–4.
13. Vergare M, Binder R, Cook I, et al. Psychiatric evaluation of adults. 2nd edition. Washington, DC: American Psychiatric Association; 2006. p. 1–62.
14. Adams P, Nielson H. Evidence based practice: decreasing psychiatric revisits to the emergency department. Issues Ment Health Nurs 2012;33(8):536–43.
15. Okafor M, Wrenn G, Ede V, et al. Improving quality of emergency care through integration of mental health. Community Ment Health J 2015;52(3):332–42.
16. Zun L. Care of psychiatric patients: the challenge to emergency physicians. West J Emerg Med 2016;17(2):173–6.
17. Stowell K, Florence P, Harman H, et al. Psychiatric evaluation of the agitated patient: consensus statement of the American Association for Emergency Psychiatry Project BETA Psychiatric Evaluation Workgroup. West J Emerg Med 2012;13(1):11–6.
18. Saldanha C. Legal issues in emergency psychiatry. In: Glick R, Berlin J, Fishkind A, et al, editors. Emergency psychiatry: principles and practice. Philadelphia: Lippincott Williams & Wilkins; 2008. p. 371–80.
19. Manton A. Care of the psychiatric patient in the emergency department 2013. Available at: Ena.org https://www.ena.org/docs/default-source/resource-library/practice-resources/white-papers/care-of-psychiatric-patient-in-the-ed.pdf?sfvrsn=3fc76cda_4. Accessed October 9, 2018.
20. Folstein M, Folstein S, McHugh P. "Mini-mental state": a practical method for grading the cognitive state of patients for the clinician. J Psychiatr Res 1975;12(3):189–98.
21. Halter M. Varcarolis' Foundations of psychiatric-mental health nursing. 8th edition. St Louis (MO): Elsevier; 2018. p. 509–10.
22. Battaglia J. Pharmacological management of acute agitation. Drugs 2005;65:1207–22.
23. Wilson MP, Pepper D, Currier GW, et al. The psychopharmacology of agitation: consensus statement of the American Association for Emergency Psychiatry Project BETA Psychopharmacology Workgroup. West J Emerg Med 2012;13(1):26–34.

24. Nicks B, Manthey D. The impact of psychiatric patient boarding in Emergency Departments. Emerg Med Int 2012;2012:360308.
25. Crisis in the Emergency Department: removing barriers to timely and appropriate mental health treatment. 2015. Available at: http://www.ssvms.org/PORTALS/7/assets/pdf/ssvms-crisis_in_the_emergency_dept.pdf. Accessed November 29, 2018.

Nurse Practitioners Improving Emergency Department Quality and Patient Outcomes

Leanne H. Fowler, DNP, MBA, AGACNP-BC, CNE[a],*,
Jessica Landry, DNP, FNP-C[a], Melissa F. Nunn, MSN, CPNP-PC[b]

KEYWORDS

• Emergency department • Nurse practitioner • ED outcomes • NP quality

KEY POINTS

- There are five types of nurse practitioners (NPs) qualified to work in emergency department (ED) settings: adult-gerontology acute care NP, adult-gerontology primary care NP, pediatric acute care NP, pediatric primary care NP, and primary care family NP.
- Research suggests that NPs practicing in ED settings improve ED quality metrics and patient outcomes.
- Studies demonstrate that NPs practicing in ED settings increase patient satisfaction, reduce door-to-provider time, reduce diagnostic test utilization, and reduce rates of patients leaving without being seen by a health care provider.
- NPs practicing in ED settings improve a variety of national quality metrics, ultimately improving the timeliness, efficiency, effectiveness, and quality of care.

In busy emergency departments (ED), efficacy and performance are measured through certain health care metrics. In the ED, common metrics include a patient's length of stay (LOS) and time to treatment. Patient LOS is the time between check-in to discharge or admission. Time to treatment is the time between checking in to the ED until assessment by a medical provider (eg, nurse practitioner [NP], physician's assistant, or physician). Other outcomes measured in the ED include patient satisfaction and financial outcomes, such as cost and expenditures.

Through clinical processes, such as "door-to-balloon" protocols for acute coronary events, many patient outcomes are measured in the ED. LOS metrics can assist ED

Disclosure Statement: The authors have nothing to disclose.
[a] LSU Health New Orleans School of Nursing, 1900 Gravier Street, New Orleans, LA 70112, USA;
[b] Children's Hospital New Orleans, LSU Health New Orleans School of Nursing, 200 Henry Clay Avenue, New Orleans, LA 70118, USA
* Corresponding author.
E-mail address: lfowle@lsuhsc.edu

Crit Care Nurs Clin N Am 31 (2019) 237–247
https://doi.org/10.1016/j.cnc.2019.02.010
0899-5885/19/© 2019 Elsevier Inc. All rights reserved.

administrators to capture comprehensive experiences for patients and can also justify the use of emergency services.[1] As patients' ED use increases, there is an increased financial burden on the health care system to effectively and efficiently manage these patients. ED overcrowding can lead to longer LOS, decreased patient satisfaction, and decreased provider productivity.[2] Such overcrowding is also linked with delays in care, along with increased short-term mortality and morbidity.[3]

In addition, to the patient experience, health care metrics can also be tied to hospital reimbursement. The Centers for Medicare and Medicaid Services target not only hospital-wide and clinic initiatives, but EDs, for quality, cost-effective care. Centers for Medicare and Medicaid Services targeted ED outcomes include patient leaving before being seen, door to diagnostic evaluation, median time from ED arrival to discharge or admission, and time from admission decision to ED departure for admitted patients. The utilization of certain metrics, such as LOS and time to treatment, is directly related to hospital reimbursement.

NPs are advanced practice registered nurses qualified to improve outcomes related to increased ED utilization. The education and training of acute and primary care NPs includes an emphasis on quality improvement, navigating a quickly evolving health care system, and collaborating with an interprofessional health care team. Trending ED metrics can demonstrate how ED NPs improve LOS, delays in treatment, patient satisfaction, and cost-effectiveness.

This article provides background information on the types of NPs that work in the ED, ED settings that NPs practice, and state of the science on NP-related patient outcomes in the ED setting.

TYPES OF NURSE PRACTITIONERS IN THE EMERGENCY DEPARTMENT

The NP role was initiated more than 50 years ago. Because of this young age, many health care personnel and clinicians are unfamiliar with their level of education and training, which continues to evolve and expand in response to a rapidly evolving health care delivery system. NPs are advanced practice registered nurses with master's or doctoral level education who blend their nursing expertise with the advanced nursing functions of prevention, diagnosis, and management of disease. NPs have an added emphasis in their education to approach each patient (with or without disease) through a comprehensive lens focusing on disease prevention and management for individuals and families.[4] NP competencies and education has evolved over the last 50 years since the role's inception. Currently, there are eight types of NPs with a population-specific focus (Table 1) who are educated at the master's or doctoral level. Of the eight types of NPs, there are five types of NPs that may work in ED settings including those nationally board-certified as an adult-gerontology acute care NP, adult-gerontology primary care NP, pediatric acute care NP, pediatric primary care NP, or primary care family NP. Regardless of the degree program or NP population-focus, there are common core competencies (Table 2) every NP must attain during their formal graduate education and before certification and licensure.[5] Responsive to the demands of current and projected health care trends, NPs entry-to-practice education is planned to transition to the Doctor of Nursing Practice degree by year 2025.[6,7]

Acute care NPs, adult-gerontology, and pediatric population-foci are educated and trained to care for patients with acute, critical, or complex chronic physical and mental illness in diverse care settings. Primary care NP competencies, for adult-gerontology, family, and pediatric population-foci, focus on preventative health care, episodic/acute illness, and chronic illness management. Primary care NP education has great

Table 1
Population-focused nurse practitioners

NP Population-Foci	Description
Acute care NPs	Emphasis on complex acute, chronic, and critical illness. Health promotion and the chronic use of medical devices is included.
Primary care NPs	Emphasis on preventative health, long-term management of chronic disease, and minor acute illness.
Adult-gerontology primary care	Manages the acute or primary care young adult (13 y and older), adult, and older adult.
Neonatal	Manages the acute care neonate up to 2 y old.
Pediatric	Manages the acute or primary care newborn to young adult patient.
Family	Manages the primary care patient and family across the lifespan: birth to older adult and inclusive of gender health.
Psychiatric-mental health	Manages the primary care patient and family across the lifespan.
Women's/gender health	Manages the primary care adolescent/young adult for gender-specific health.

Data from Adult-Gerontology NP Competencies Work Group. Adult-gerontology, acute care, and primary care NP competencies. 2016. Available at: https://cdn.ymaws.com/www.nonpf.org/resource/resmgr/competencies/NP_Adult_Geri_competencies_4.pdf; and Population-Focused Competencies Task Force. Population-focused nurse practitioners competencies. 2013. Available at: https://cdn.ymaws.com/www.nonpf.org/resource/resmgr/Competencies/CompilationPopFocusComps2013.pdf. Accessed January 5, 2019.

emphasis on disease prevention, chronic disease management, and minor acute illness management. There are acute care and primary care adult-gerontology NP population-focused competencies. Adult-gerontology NPs care for the young adult (13 years and older), adult, and older adult (60 years and older). There are also acute and primary care pediatric NP competencies. Pediatric NPs focus on caring for children from birth to young adulthood experiencing acute, critical, or complex medical or mental illness respective to the acute or primary care population-focus. The primary care family NP competencies focus on the education and training needed to care for individuals and families across the entire life span with emphasis on family-centered care. This population focus often refers to their competencies spanning the care of individuals and families "from the womb to the tomb" and differs from other primary care NP foci in the breadth of education and training to care for pediatric, adult, and gender-specific health promotion and disease management.[8–10]

TYPES OF EMERGENCY DEPARTMENT SETTINGS FOR NURSE PRACTITIONER PRACTICE
Academic Setting

NPs deliver high-quality, effective, and safe health care to various patient populations across a wide range of health care settings.[11] In the academic hospital setting, NPs in the ED are expected to function in a fast-paced, high-stress workplace that requires interprofessional relationships and collaboration. In this type of workplace, dynamic and blurred professional lines can lead to tension unless roles and expectations of team members are clearly defined and communicated.[12]

Table 2
Core competency areas for nurse practitioners

Competency Area	Emphasis
Scientific foundation	The application, analysis, and translation of fundamental sciences, humanities, and nursing knowledge.
Leadership	The use of reflective thinking, communication skills, and collaborative engagement with interprofessional teams and professional organizations.
Quality	The evaluation of the relationship organizational processes has with clinical practice to promote a culture of safety, high quality, and translation of the best research.
Practice inquiry	The generation, application, analysis, translation, and dissemination of knowledge into clinical practice.
Technology and information literacy	The use of and integration of information technology literacy and systems to improve practice and patient outcomes.
Policy	The application and analysis of ethical, legal, and social factors that influence policy and practice. Also, the role of advocacy for policies that influence practice.
Health delivery system	The analysis and evaluation of health care delivery systems, organizations, and environments that impact the needs of culturally diverse populations and the delivery of care.
Ethics	The integration of ethical principles in decision making and evaluation of the consequences of decisions.
Independent practice	The demonstration of patient-centered, culturally centered, and spiritually centered, accountable, collaborative, high-quality, efficient, and competent care to the full scope of practice. The education of professional and lay caregivers and coordination of health care services, teams, and transition of care.

Data from National Organization of Nurse Practitioner Faculties. Nurse practitioner core competencies content. Available at: https://www.nonpf.org/resource/resmgr/competencies/2017_NPCoreComps_with_Curric.pdf. Accessed January 5, 2019.

Private Institutions

Issues related to hospital ED quality and performance are particularly important to privately managed institutions and is challenging to even the best resourced facilities.[13–15] Overcrowding, frequently seen in urban EDs, is burdensome for those facilities aiming to meet or exceed benchmarks. In an attempt to improve throughput, two strategies have been found to be successful: a designated NP for fast track and/or a designated NP for triage. Fast-track units have been shown to streamline patients presenting with less emergent illnesses and injuries and NPs have been shown to be able to consistently provide efficient and quality care.[16] Fast-track patients with an Emergency Severity Index Scale (ESI) of four or five are seen by the NP independently or with physician collaboration if needed (**Table 3**).

Having a designated NP in the triage bay with the registered nurse is another measure to ensure faster door-to-provider times.[14] Having an NP see the patient at their time of arrival has several benefits: (1) the patient is examined by a provider immediately (more accurate ESI level assignment), (2) decreased number of patients leaving without being seen by a provider, (3) communication to the patient that an ED is committed to providing them immediate care regardless of the complaint (patient satisfaction), (4) decreased LOS if orders are placed at the time of arrival versus after

Table 3		
Emergency Severity Index (ESI) scale		
ESI Level	**Definition**	**Example**
Level 1	Life threatening condition/ loss of life or limb	Trauma Respiratory arrest Decompensated STEMI
Level 2	Emergency	NSTEMI Ischemic stroke Intracranial hemorrhage
Level 3	Urgent condition	Abdominal pain Moderate-severe epistaxis
Level 4 (fast track)	Less urgent conditions	Uncomplicated laceration Uncomplicated abscess Cough/influenza
Level 5 (fast track)	Nonurgent conditions	Prescription refill Suture/staple removal

Abbreviations: NSTEMI, non–ST-segment elevation myocardial infarction; STEMI, ST-segment elevation myocardial infarction.

Data from Gilboy N, Tanabe P, Travers D, et al. Emergency Severity Index (ESI): a triage tool for emergency department care implementation handbook. Available at: https://www.ahrq.gov/sites/default/files/wysiwyg/professionals/systems/hospital/esi/esihandbk.pdf. Accessed January 5, 2019.

the patient is roomed (eg, abdominal pain orders placed initially, patient waits 45 minutes to be roomed, by the time the patient is roomed, laboratory and/or imaging studies are ready for review), and (5) improved efficiency and throughput.[13,14]

Rural Hospitals

EDs in rural setting have unique challenges, such as a limited number of providers on staff at a given time. Physicians may practice as a single provider in these institutions and not have double coverage or available backup. When a critical patient presents to these types of facilities, the single provider's time may be consumed for long periods while other patients wait for medical attention. Utilization of an NP in rural EDs can better serve rural communities. In a study involving a rural urgent care staffed by NPs, it was noted that patients had high levels of satisfaction, lower total LOS, believed they had enough time to communicate their problems and discuss after care, and 97% believed that the quality of the emergency NP was of a high standard.[17]

STATE OF THE SCIENCE ON NURSE PRACTITIONERS IMPROVING PATIENT OUTCOMES IN EMERGENCY DEPARTMENTS
Literature Review

A literature search was conducted using the databases of EBSCOhost and CINAHL. Keywords included: "emergency department," "nurse practitioner," "outcomes," "quality," "waiting times," "cost effective," and "efficacy." Inclusion criteria were studies from peer reviewed academic journal articles available in English and full text published from 2013 to 2019. A total of 619 articles met inclusion criteria. Eight articles were selected for review of content and are discussed next. Of the studies selected, there were four systematic reviews, one randomized controlled trial (RCT), one qualitative study, one descriptive study, and one longitudinal cohort study. **Table 4** provides individual article findings.

Table 4
Summary of findings

Author	Type of Study	Findings/NP Outcomes
Roche et al,[13] 2017	Longitudinal cohort study 61 patients with chest pain who presented to rural ED with chest pain were evaluated from 2014 to 2016 were included in cohort 41 patients with suspected or confirmed acute coronary syndrome were identified Compared difference in care of NP with ED physician	Results indicated NPs showed high adherence to recommended guidelines in the management of chest pain 91.7% NPs achieved diagnostic accuracy on electrocardiogram compared with usual care at 82.8% Effective and reasonable waiting times Effective and reasonable length of stay Excellent patient outcomes 100% patients seen by NP were either satisfied or highly satisfied
McDevitt and Melby,[17] 2014	Descriptive study Case note review and survey design with one open-ended exploratory question Patient self-completed questionnaire Data extraction tool to survey patients' case notes retrospectively	NPs studied showed to deliver safe care Showed to deliver quality care Demonstrated high level of patient satisfaction Allowed adequate consultation time with patients Embraced a holistic approach Provided injury and health promotion education Used clear communication
Li et al,[19] 2013	Cross-sectional qualitative study Performed across two large academic institutions Involved physicians, nurses, administrators, and NPs	NPs perceived to be leaders in embracing a preventative paradigm ED staff interviewed had overall positive and affirming attitudes toward NP practice Nurses believed NPs saw patients quickly and greatly improved the care in the fast-tract setting NPs were role-models to other nurses Physicians believed NPs spent more time explaining care to patients Physicians believed the presence of the NP allowed them to spend more time with higher acuity patients NP care was believed to be more holistic in nature
Begaz et al,[14] 2017	Prospective randomized controlled trial Secondary analysis of data of waiting room diagnostic testing 770 patients had studies ordered from waiting rooms The number of tests and length of stay were compared between having a physician in triage and an NP in triage	NPs ordered fewer diagnostic tests than physicians Having a physician in triage prolonged length of stay NP use in triage was greatly supported

(continued on next page)

Table 4 *(continued)*		
Author	**Type of Study**	**Findings/NP Outcomes**
Stanik-Hutt et al,[20] 2013	Systematic review Data used from 37 of 27,993 articles Articles from 1990 to 2009 11 outcomes reviewed	NPs demonstrated high-quality health care Improved patient safety Effectively managed care As effective as physicians in the management of glucose control As effective as physicians in the management of blood pressure control Patients reported high levels of satisfaction
Jennings et al,[21] 2015	Systematic review 14 of 1013 studies were included 4 databases searched from 2006 to 2013	NPs positively affect patient satisfaction Decreased waiting times High overall quality of care No difference in care (outcomes) were determined when compared with physician Shown to be cost-effective
Woo et al,[11] 2017	Systematic review Searched 9 databases Articles from 2006 to 2016 15 studies chosen for appraisal Data extracted using standardized tools	NP effectively managed minor injuries Decreased length of stay Worked well with interdisciplinary team Conducted appropriate discharge planning Provided patient education Worked well independently
Martin-Misener et al,[18] 2018	Systematic review Used randomized controlled trials from 1980 to 2015 Included 11 trials for appraisal Searched 10 databases Included hand searches	NPs had equivalent or better patient outcomes than physicians NPs were cost-effective care providers Spent 4.1 min longer with patients Patients reported they were educated regarding their illness, management, and aftercare

Synopsis of Literature

In a systematic review by Woo and colleagues,[11] 15 studies published between 2006 and 2016 were examined and the results demonstrated the impact of NPs on quality care, patient satisfaction, and cost-effectiveness in the emergency and critical settings. It was determined that NP professional performance directly improved patient outcomes.[11] This review determined that NPs increased patient access to emergency care and were shown to be effectively used as an integral part of the health care team. The authors included studies that showed the NP managed injuries, decreased total LOS, worked with a multidisciplinary team, conducted effective discharge planning, provided patient education, and worked independently.[11] Other studies in the review reported that patient satisfaction scores improved with NP care, particularly when the NP was used in the fast-track setting. The systematic review showed that NPs ordered appropriate medications, diagnostic testing, and decreased the number of patients leaving the ED without being seen. Lastly, the authors determined that NPs decreased door-to-needle time, overall wait times, number of patients who left without being seen, staffing costs, and patient mortality.[11]

In a 2018 systematic review, the authors included studies that examined the care delivered by NPs published from 1980 to 2015.[18] Eleven RCTs were included and demonstrated trends that care provided by NPs were associated with higher levels of patient satisfaction and demonstrated patient health outcomes comparable with that of a physician. The NPs were shown to spend an average of 4.1 minutes longer with patients, and in return, patients reported they were educated well on their illness, symptom management, and follow-up care.[18] This systematic review determined that NPs had lower mean health services cost per consultation when compared with a physician deeming NPs were cost-effective.

A cross-sectional qualitative study with ED administrators, physicians, NPs, and nurses in various EDs determined overall positive and affirming attitudes toward NPs and the care they provide.[19] Nurses reported that after the addition of NPs in the ED, patients were seen quicker and NPs were particularly effective in the fast-track area. They also described NPs as positive role models for nurses. ED administrators reported that addition of NPs to the team positively affected work relationships and the independent role of the NP created a unique work environment. ED physicians reported that NP's patient interactions were similar to that of physician interactions; however, NPs spent more time with patients and provided better explanations about illness and aftercare.[19] Another ED physician reported feeling more freedom to concentrate on the higher acuity patients because the NPs handled those patients less acute and this allowed more time to focus on the sickest. Of the NPs interviewed, one described care by the NP to be more holistic and that NPs look for other solutions to problems (eg, nonpharmacologic approaches).

In a systematic review focused on quality and effectiveness of care provided by NPs from 1990 to 2009, it was determined NPs provided high-quality health care, improved patient safety, and were effective in managing care.[20] The results of this systematic review showed that patient care in the ED delivered by the NP was comparable with that of the physician. Healthy children and adults with minor complaints, and patients with complex illnesses were included in the sample; NPs provided safe, high-quality, comparable care. When patients were queried about their perceptions of care, they consistently reported high satisfaction rates with NP care and management. NPs were also shown to impact patient safety outcomes. Safety issues, such as medication errors, falls, infections, and skin issues, were not found to increase. NPs were shown to be as effective as physicians in the management of blood pressure, glucose control, hepatitis C, human immunodeficiency virus, heart failure, and cystic fibrosis.[20]

In a secondary analysis of data from a prospective RCT focused on the number of diagnostic tests ordered by the NP as compared with the emergency physician in the triage area, it was determined that NPs ordered fewer diagnostic tests.[14] Results showed that patients screened by physicians had a longer ED LOS because of ordering more tests initially. This study suggested that when there was an NP in triage, LOS was shorter, and throughput was improved, further supporting the role of the NP in the ED.

A systematic review of studies between 2006 and 2013 on the impact of NP services on quality of care, satisfaction, and wait times in the ED demonstrated positive results.[21] Fourteen studies were appraised, and findings demonstrated NPs provided effective quality care and no significant difference was seen when care was compared with that of the physician alone. Patients reported satisfaction with their care and reduced wait times were seen with NP delivery of care. NPs were determined to decrease LOS, time to disposition, and improve overall health outcomes.[21] In included studies, wait times improved by 19 minutes, and satisfaction was 68% for NPs compared with 50% for physicians.[21] This systematic review supports that NPs were cost-effective in the ED, but more RCTs are needed to better quantify patient outcomes.

A descriptive study conducted in a rural urgent care setting suggested NPs demonstrated clinically safe and effective practice.[17] One overarching theme in this study was patient self-report of high satisfaction with their care. Although the concept of satisfaction is subjective, it is an important outcome to assess because less satisfied patients can provide evidence for improvement. Some of the factors found to influence patient satisfaction were the patient's expectation of the visit, their overall perception of care, age, and possibly demographics.[17] Regardless of these factors, NPs produced high levels of satisfaction. NPs were also perceived by patients to possess thoroughness with their practice; spent more time with examination; and produced high standard, clear documentation. NPs had reduced actual and patient perceived wait times, ordered appropriate referrals, used clear communication, used a holistic approach, allowed adequate time for consultation with the patient, and provided injury advice and health promotion education.[17]

In a multisite prospective longitudinal nested cohort study, the effectiveness of NP services to patients presenting to rural hospitals with chest pain was examined.[13] This study aimed to determine the safety, quality, and effectiveness of the care by NPs in the ED. NPs consistently prescribed and ordered diagnostic tests in accordance with current recommended guidelines. Findings also demonstrated that NPs achieved 91.7% diagnostic accuracy of electrocardiograph interpretation compared with standard care of 82.8%.[13] Service indicators, such as wait times and LOS, were also improved, and 91.5% of patients reported being "highly satisfied," whereas 8.5% reported they were "satisfied" with their care.[13]

Discussion

The literature review exposed several themes when considering the care NPs provide for patients in the ED. NPs increased patient satisfaction, reduced wait times, demonstrated care comparable with physicians, spent more time with patients, adhered to high standard documentation, followed current recommended guidelines, and worked well in teams.[11,17,18,21] More evidence is needed to fully quantify the cost-effectiveness of NPs in the ED.[22] A gap in the literature exists in the evidence of how pediatric NPs in a pediatric ED affect patient outcomes specifically.[23]

The care provided by an NP was consistent internationally, in urban and rural settings, in academic and private institutions, and in acute and urgent settings.[11,17,20] NP care was also consistent with different populations and patient acuities across the lifespan. NPs were shown to effectively manage healthy subjects with minor illnesses or injuries and those with complex comorbid conditions.[12,13,20]

There has been a rapid uptake of NPs in the ED and challenges still exist affecting NP practice.[12,24] Some states allow NPs to practice at their full scope as others have restrictions, this can lead to wide variations in actual practice.[12] Another consideration is that some aspects of the emergency NP workload may not always be visible and could be underrepresented. One-quarter of emergency NP patient encounters are patients presenting with highly complex conditions.[25] NPs in ED settings are managing patients beyond minor injury and illness and must ensure competence, capability, and that they remain within their scope of practice.[25] NPs also reported that their work environments directly affected their ability to practice within their scope.[26]

Another factor that may affect outcomes is how the emergency NP views their role within the department. In a qualitative study where NPs were surveyed, one of the themes was that NPs have stress regarding role expansion and the future of their role in the ED.[27] Role development is an ongoing and ever-changing factor and directly tied to job satisfaction, successful teamwork, and patient outcomes.[25]

Overcrowding continues to be an issue in EDs around the globe. The problem begins when more patients are taken into the ED at one time than are discharged. Several strategies can be used to improve the situation of overcrowding including development of holding units within the ED (requires construction), creating political changes to increase resources, or simply by improving discharge timing.[14] NPs were consistently shown to decrease LOS, which includes moving patients out of the ED in a timely manner.[11,21]

SUMMARY

NP utilization in the ED is a promising solution to increased patient numbers. NPs are qualified to provide safe, efficient, high-quality care in the ED and were proven to earn equivalent, if not higher, patient satisfaction ratings. Through further exposure in EDs and continued dialogues with other health care providers, NPs are an integral part of the patient care team for a well-functioning emergency department. Further research on NP's impact on ED patient outcomes and quality with higher acuity ED patients is needed.

REFERENCES

1. Agency for Healthcare Research and Quality [AHRQ]. Section 3. Measuring emergency department performance. Available at: http://www.ahrq.gov/research/findings/final-reports/ptflow/section3.html. Accessed January 5, 2019.
2. Imperato J, Morris DS, Sanchez LD, et al. Improving patient satisfaction by adding a physician in triage. J Hosp Adm 2013;3:7–13.
3. Chang AM, Cohen DJ, Lin A, et al. Hospital strategies for reducing emergency department crowding: a mixed-methods study. Ann Emerg Med 2018;71:497–505.
4. American Association of Nurse Practitioners [AANP]. What's a nurse practitioner (NP)?. Available at: https://www.aanp.org/about/all-about-nps/whats-a-nurse-practitioner. Accessed January 5, 2019.
5. National Organization of Nurse Practitioner Faculties [NONPF]. Nurse practitioner core competencies content. Washington, DC: NONPF; 2017.
6. National Organizations of Nurse Practitioner Faculties [NONPF]. NONPF DNP statement may 2018. NONPF; 2018. Available at: https://www.nonpf.org/news/400012/NONPF-DNP-Statement-May-2018.htm. Accessed January 1 2019.
7. American Association of Colleges of Nursing [AACN]. Adult-gerontology acute care and primary care NP competencies. Washington, DC: AACN; 2016.
8. National Organization of Nurse Practitioner Faculties [NONPF]. Population-focused nurse practitioner competencies. Washington, DC: NONPF; 2013.
9. American Association of Colleges of Nursing [AACN]. The essentials of doctoral education for advanced nursing practice 2006. Available at: https://www.aacnnursing.org/Portals/42/Publications/DNPEssentials.pdf. Accessed January 5 2019.
10. American Association of Colleges of Nursing [AACN]. The essentials of Master's education in nursing 2011. Available at: https://www.aacnnursing.org/Portals/42/Publications/MastersEssentials11.pdf. Accessed January 6 2019.
11. Woo BFY, Lee JXY, Tam WWS. The impact of the advanced practice nursing role on quality of care, clinical outcomes, patient satisfaction, and cost in the

emergency and critical care settings: a systematic review. Hum Resour Health 2017;15:1–22.

12. Poghosyan DB, Knutson AR. Nurse practitioner role, independent practice, and teamwork in primary care. J Nurse Pract 2014;10:472–9.

13. Roche TE, Gardner G, Jack L. The effectiveness of emergency nurse practitioner service in the management of patients presenting to rural hospitals with chest pain: a multisite prospective longitudinal nested cohort study. BMC Health Serv Res 2017;17:1–14.

14. Begaz T, Elashoff D, Grogan TR, et al. Differences in test ordering between nurse practitioners and attending emergency physicians when acting as provider in triage. Am J Emerg Med 2017;35:1426–9.

15. Chan SW, Cheung NK, Graham CA, et al. Strategies and solutions to alleviate access block and overcrowding in emergency departments. Hong Kong Med J 2015;21:345–52.

16. Doetzel JA, Rankin JA, Then KL. Nurse practitioners in the emergency department: barriers and facilitators for role implementation. Adv Emerg Nurs J 2016; 38:43–55.

17. McDevitt J, Melby V. An evaluation of the quality of emergency nurse practitioner services for patients presenting with minor injuries to one rural urgent care center in the UK: a descriptive study. J Clin Nurs 2014;24:523–35.

18. Martin-Misener R, Harbman P, Donald F, et al. Cost-effectiveness of nurse practitioners in primary and specialized ambulatory care: systematic review. BMJ Open 2018;5:1–14.

19. Li J, Westbrook J, Callen J, et al. The impact of nurse practitioners on care delivery in the emergency department: a multiple perspectives approach. BMC Health Serv Res 2013;13:356.

20. Stanik-Hutt J, Newhouse RP, White K, et al. The quality and effectiveness of care provided by nurse practitioners. J Nurse Pract 2013;9:492–500e.

21. Jennings N, Clifford S, Fox A, et al. The impact of nurse practitioner services on cost, quality of care, satisfaction and waiting times in the emergency department: a systematic review. Int J Nurs Stud 2015;52:421–35.

22. Craswell A, Dwyer T, Rossi D, et al. Cost-effectiveness of nurse practitioner led regional titration service for heart failure patients. J Nurse Pract 2018;14:105–11.

23. Rutledge TR, Merritt LS. Pediatric nurse practitioners in the emergency department: implications for education and research. J Pediatr Health Care 2017;31: 729–33.

24. Jennings N, Gardner G, O'Reilly G. A protocol for a pragmatic randomized controlled trial evaluating outcomes of emergency nurse practitioner services. J Adv Nurs 2014;70:2140–8.

25. Lutze M, Fry M, Mullen G, et al. Highlighting the invisible work of emergency nurse practitioners. J Nurse Pract 2018;14:26–32.

26. Poghosyan L, Nannini A, Smaldone A, et al. Revisiting scope of practice facilitators and barrier for primary care nurse practitioners: a qualitative investigation. Policy Polit Nurs Pract 2013;10:6–15.

27. Lloyd-Rees J. How emergency nurse practitioners view their role within the emergency department: a qualitative study. Int Emerg Nurs 2016;24:46–53.

Hospitals Providing Temporary Emergency Department Services in Alternative Care Settings After Hurricane Sandy

Anne Reid Griffin, MPH, BSN, RN[a],*, Alicia R. Gable, MPH[a],
Claudia Der-Martirosian, PhD[a], Aram Dobalian, PhD, JD, MPH[a,b]

KEYWORDS

- Disaster • Hospital evacuation • Emergency departments • Patient care • Veterans
- Vulnerable populations

KEY POINTS

- When hospitals close because of major disasters, those who are most vulnerable often do not evacuate and continue to need emergent care.
- Research is needed to inform practical guidance for hospitals to provide temporary emergency services in alterative care settings.
- Meanwhile, hospital planners should anticipate that many of their most vulnerable patients will continue to need care and viable solutions should be considered for immediate and long-term needs.

INTRODUCTION

Hurricane Sandy wreaked havoc on New York City on October 29, 2012. The massive flood surge impacted 51 square miles across the 5 New York City Boroughs—Manhattan, The Bronx, Queens, Brooklyn, and Staten Island. Severe flash flooding and extensive damage to critical infrastructure resulted in widespread power outages, the elimination of mass transit, limited access to highways, and gas shortages. The US Department of Veterans Affairs (VA) New York Harbor Healthcare System (NYHHS)

Disclosure Statement: The authors have nothing to disclose.
[a] Veterans Emergency Management Evaluation Center, US Department of Veterans Affairs, 16111 Plummer Street, MS-152, North Hills, CA 91343, USA; [b] Division of Health Systems Management and Policy, The University of Memphis School of Public Health, Memphis, TN 38152, USA
* Corresponding author.
E-mail address: anne.griffin@va.gov

evacuated their inpatient and outpatient facilities ahead of the storm. VA outpatient services resumed 5 months later and the inpatient and emergency department (ED) reopened 7 months later. New York University Hospital Langone Medical Center (NYU) and Bellevue Medical Center both evacuated during the storm because of storm damage. NYU resumed inpatient services 2 months later and their ED reopened 18 months later. Bellevue resumed their inpatient service and ED just over 3 months later. Located within 2 miles of each other, these 3 hospitals collectively provided 500 ED visits per day before the storm.[1]

News reports described what happened after the extended closure of the 3 EDs in lower Manhattan after Hurricane Sandy. The 4 hospitals that received the majority of surge from the evacuated hospitals reported a 20% increase in ED volume,[2] because they inherited ED patients needing care for chronic medical conditions, influenza, pharmaceuticals, and methadone dosing.[2] Beth Israel was the only remaining open hospital in lower Manhattan and had patients forming lines out the door. Their ED census increased from 300 per day to as many as 500 per day during the week that followed the storm.[3] In particular, they experienced a spike in the volume of oxygen-dependent patients and patients needing dialysis and medication refills.[4] Weill Cornell Medical Center, the closest trauma center to Bellevue, experienced a 25% increase in emergency room visits.[5] New York Presbyterian Hospital described caring for patients in methadone withdrawal because as many as 90% of the opiate treatment programs in the impacted area were not operating after the storm.[5]

Meanwhile, many committed professionals in the community rallied to support the health needs of those sheltering in Manhattan for months after the storm. The North Shore Long Island Jewish Health System targeted New York's hardest hit communities by launching mobile health units within 2 to 3 weeks of the storm.[6] The State Department of Health along with New York City organized 11 mobile primary care units that canvased impacted areas and provided 4000 visits. The National Guard provided care to 600 people in their home and the Visiting Nurse Service of New York provided 1100 assessments.[7]

All 3 hospitals that evacuated (NYU, Bellevue, and VA NYHHS) took steps to address the unmet needs of their patients. For example, Lee and colleagues[1] described the incremental steps Bellevue Hospital took to rebuild emergency care after Hurricane Sandy. Within 3 weeks of the hurricane, 24-hour urgent care services were resumed. A freestanding, nonambulance receiving ED followed 3 weeks later. With those 2 steps, Bellevue was providing care for almost one-half of its usual ED volume. In tandem, primary and specialty care reopened. Within another 2 weeks, the ED was designated as a 911 receiving facility, which helped to mitigate high ambulance volume and normalize the demand on neighboring hospitals. Despite the continued hospital closure, their ED was providing 77% of its prehurricane care.[1]

Caspers and colleagues[8] described the strategies NYU took to remove strain on Beth Israel and restore their acute care services. They opened an on-campus urgent care center and implemented their first ED-run Observation Service (EDOS) while their ED remained closed. The authors conducted a retrospective cohort study of all patients placed in the EDOS after a visit to the urgent care and identified diagnoses, clinical protocols, selection criteria, and performance metrics. The authors concluded that a diverse group of patients presenting to an urgent care center after the destruction of an ED by a disaster can be cared for in an EDOS, regardless of a physical ED.[8]

The primary purpose of this article is to document how the VA cared for vulnerable veterans who did not evacuate from lower Manhattan after Hurricane Sandy, while the Manhattan Veterans Affairs Medical Center (VAMC), including the ED, was closed for an extended period owing to flooding damage sustained from the hurricane.

METHODS

This was a nonexperimental, phenomenological study of the lived experience of senior clinicians, administrators, and ancillary/operations managers from NYHHS as well as administrators and emergency managers from the administrate area of the Veteran Integrated Services Network (VISN 3), who participated in the campus evacuation 1 day before Hurricane Sandy.

The interview guide was developed from a prior study examining VA nursing home evacuations after Hurricanes Katrina and Rita,[9] a hospital evacuation tool published by Schultz and colleagues,[4] and the hospital evacuation literature.[10–13] The primary focus of the study was the decision to evacuate the hospital in advance of Hurricane Sandy. The interview guide includes questions about prior disaster response experience, participation in disaster preparedness planning and exercises, preparations and planning in the days leading up to the event, the evacuation decision process, and the operations and logistics of the evacuation. Open-ended questions were constructed to elicit responses in a conversational style and to encourage participants to expand on their experiences. The questions pertaining to the topic of this article include the following.

1. What was done to ensure continuity of care surrounding the evacuation?
2. What was the single most important unanticipated problem that could have had negative consequences for either patient care or movement?

The senior author and another member of the research team conducted individual interviews in person or over the telephone 3 months after the evacuation while the Manhattan campus was still formally closed. All interviews were audio recorded and transcribed. Participants were advised that the study was voluntary and they could refuse to participate at any time or refuse to answer any question. The Institutional Review Board of the VA Greater Los Angeles Healthcare System approved this study.

Data Analysis

Interview transcripts were analyzed using Atlas.ti (Version 7.1.6, Scientific Software Development GmbH, Berlin, Germany). Deductive codes were based on the interview guide as well as supporting literature. Inductive codes were based on the interview data. Two authors independently coded each transcript and reconciled coding differences through discussion.

RESULTS

A convenience sampling approach was used to identify and invite 43 VA staff from the NYHHS and VISN 3. Of those, 29 staff members agreed, 6 refused, and 8 did not respond to the invitation. The interview sample included 12 senior clinicians, 7 administrators, 7 ancillary/operations managers, and 3 VISN administrators or emergency managers.

Themes

Vulnerable veterans remained after the hurricane and continued to need care
The safety of inpatients was the primary focus during the hospital evacuation. Although messages about the VAMC closure were disseminated to veterans via multiple channels (website, newspapers, television, radio), vulnerable veterans in lower Manhattan remained and did seek treatment from the closed VAMC after the storm.

[T]he storm was Monday. On the Tuesday after the storm, started making phone calls to patients. But I'm sure a lot of people were not reached. Some of them

probably still have not been reached, even though we've put ads and phone numbers and tried to reach everybody we could.

The Post Office shut down. The Post Office is the way we deliver a lot of medications to patients. So, a lot of people didn't get their medications exactly when they should. I think the Post Office was actually shut down for about a week. Then there was a backlog probably of at least another week or two in Manhattan in just distributing some of the mail. Obviously, it didn't get through.

I mean, there was an evacuation. Then the building was absolutely positively empty. Then after the storm, we saw that stragglers, everybody did not get the memo that the hospital was closed. People were showing up. Because they would come in and say, "What do you mean the hospital's closed? What do you mean it's not open? What do you mean there was a hurricane?" And you would realize how impaired and cut off these people were.

A lot of our patients are homeless. So, they had neither places nor necessarily telephones where they could be reached.

A creative approach was required to manage the immediate needs of veterans seeking care

Veterans continued to seek care from the closed facility, which forced the VA to develop a strategy for triage and the provision of care. Generators were arranged to power key parts of the hospital and within days the previously dark lobby had power, phones, computers, tables, and chairs.

So, it was sort of an ad hoc thing for a day or two. And the patients, what we would do is ascertain if they needed critical care. And if they did, we'd get an ambulance.

On the third or fourth day, one of the nights is when we decided to set up the lobby.

We put the tables out. We put the chairs out. I got IT to do the phones and the computers. And we realized that, since we had no fire alarm system, we really weren't bringing people in. But we also realized that people will still come to the hospital, asking questions. "What do we do next?" So we had to set up some kind of command area. So we set up a command office in that glass area there. And then the barrier was the police table. So that people could come into the lobby, but that was as far as we could let them go.

So it took some time for us to figure out where we could see patients at the other, alternate sites, and what would be best done right in the lobby here.

A creative approach was required to manage the long-term needs of veterans seeking care

Over the course of several weeks, the VA provided mobile medical vans just outside the building and assembled teams of clinicians, including an emergency physician, psychiatrist, nurse, and pharmacist. These clinicians provided triage, basic primary care, mental health care, medication refills, blood pressure monitoring, and the collection of time-sensitive laboratory specimens.

Then it became standardized that there were several clinicians in the lobby, including psychiatrists. So pretty much from that point on, we've had a psychiatrist in the lobby every day who writes refills, has had a few patients, actually had to call 911 on because they came in and were actually acutely ill. But, we've had that presence in the lobby.

For any other outpatient services, we'd have them go down to Beth Israel, which was the closest hospital that was open. But we did tell them that they could go to [VA Medical Centers in] Brooklyn or the Bronx. But remember, the subways weren't running, so that was... So most of them did not opt to do that.

We did have people deployed very quickly, I felt that our service was actually well-organized in a variety of ways and proactive, one being that we made sure that we had both homeless [services]and medical triage people located at the New York campus pretty much from the beginning to help with the triaging and resource assistance and so on, on the spot. We knew that there were going to be veterans that were just going to show up at the hospital like nothing happened and of course, they were going to be looking for help and a lot of them were elderly and it was like, we've got to have somebody there to do that.

In addition to providing clinical services, the VA presence provided an important message to the patients they serve. The VA continued to provide this level of care for 5 months.

And so that's why early on, we set up some services in the lobby...that's really been very helpful because it was a presence and besides actually rendering services, it said to our veterans, we're still here for you.

We're not here as you knew us but we're not abandoning you and we're here and we can help you and if you need prescriptions refilled, we can get that done for you. ...it was a very interesting experience to be there and to watch it and to say to folks, no, we're going to take care of you. You know, it's going to take us a little bit longer, but we're going to take care of you.

DISCUSSION

The 500 collective ED visits provided daily by NYU, Bellevue, and the Manhattan VAMC could not be ignored when the 3 hospitals in lower Manhattan closed. It is well-established that, under normal circumstances, EDs are overburdened every day as they accommodate an increasing number of patients with both complex and primary care needs.[14–18] They often care for those who are the most vulnerable—the elderly, poor, and uninsured.[19,20] In addition, evidence suggests that medically vulnerable populations often lack the ability to fully prepare for emergencies[21] and are less likely to evacuate after a disaster.[22]

The response in New York City parallels what happened in New Orleans when Charity Hospital, one of the busiest EDs in the country, closed because of Hurricane Katrina. Temporary surge hospitals or pop-up medical vans and clinics appeared in parking lots, retail spaces, arenas, and veterinary hospitals.[19] Care was provided by hospitals, the National Guard, the US Public Health Service, the American Red Cross, and the VA. Surveillance data collected from emergency treatment facilities throughout New Orleans estimated 21,673 visits for illness, injuries, medication refills, and routine follow-up care.[23]

A similar situation occurred when the 2018 Camp Fire in Paradise California forced Feather River Hospital to emergently evacuate all of their patients and staff. Blocked roads forced some doctors, nurses, paramedics, and police to return to the hospital; there, they found approximately 50 people who were unable to evacuate and needed medical care. Staff broke into the closed hospital to gather gurneys, oxygen tanks, and other equipment to provide triage and treatment from the hospital parking lot and helipad.[24,25]

Accredited hospitals prepare for disasters according to requirements and guidance from organizations such as the Centers for Medicare and Medicaid Services, The Joint Commission, the Occupational Safety and Health Administration, and the National Fire Prevention Association. Currently, there are no requirements for hospitals to prepare for ED care after a hospital evacuates. The Joint Commission acknowledged the attempts to cope with those who were ill after Hurricane Katrina[22] and noted that, as hospitals expanded their services beyond the walls of the physical organization, new challenges were presented to establish standards to guide care from alternative care sites.[22]

Thus, although hospitals are not required to provide care after an evacuation, the scenarios discussed in this article indicate that they do end up providing various levels of care. Each of the 3 New York hospitals implemented a wide range of creative and unique strategies to address the needs of patients with the resources that were available to them at the time. Bellevue methodically recreated an ED that would satisfy accreditation requirements at each incremental step. Because inpatient services were reestablished before the ED reopened, NYU established an urgent care center and EDOS in other parts of their hospital. This VA used mobile medical vans and leveraged their large network of providers.

Currently, there is no consensus about what level of care is needed and what is reasonable and feasible for hospitals to provide in the event they are forced to close their ED temporarily because of a disaster. Additionally, there is an absence of performance assessment criteria for hospital response in general.[26–29] Lazar and colleagues[26] suggest replicating a disaster situation by applying traditional health care quality metrics such as ED length of stay to outlier periods such as during a blackout to measure outcomes. In the case of a closed ED, perhaps a traditional metric could be applied to walk-ins during episodes of 911 diversion.

Hospital planners should consider the emergent medical and social needs of their patient populations and discuss viable solutions for providing care if their ED closes because of a disaster. Perhaps a study of those who have provided care in alternative settings after evacuation would yield insight, prompt discussions, and establish reasonable targets for providing ED care throughout stages of disaster recovery. Eventually, this information could serve as a consultative resource to provide practical guidance for hospital administrators about how they can best provide medical care in alternative settings after a disaster.

LIMITATIONS

The capabilities and resources of the VA cannot be generalized to non-VA organizations. For example, VA hospitals may have access to more physical and organizational resources. Similarly, hospitals like Bellevue and NYU have access to resources that would exceed those available to most community hospitals. This analysis is based on interviews that were primarily focused on preparedness planning and exercises, preparations in the days leading up to the event, the evacuation decision process, and the operations and logistics of the evacuation. The interview guide did not focus directly on ED care.

SUMMARY

This article documents how the VA cared for vulnerable veterans who did not evacuate from lower Manhattan after Hurricane Sandy, while the entire Manhattan VAMC was closed for an extended period owing to damage from flooding. The experience of this VA and 2 non-VA hospitals in Manhattan that closed after Hurricane Sandy highlight how vulnerable patients in the community continued to need care. Given hospital preparedness planning efforts focus primarily on sheltering in place and evacuation, research is needed to identify lessons learned from how hospitals provided temporary ED services in alternative settings to inform practical guidance for hospital administrators. Meanwhile, hospital planners should anticipate that many of their most vulnerable patients will continue to need ED care, and viable solutions should be considered.

ACKNOWLEDGMENTS

This material is based upon work supported by the U.S. Department of Veterans Affairs. The views expressed in this article are those of the authors and do not necessarily reflect the position or policy of the Department of Veterans Affairs or the U.S. government.

REFERENCES

1. Lee DC, Smith SW, McStay CM, et al. Rebuilding emergency care after Hurricane Sandy. Disaster Med Public Health Prep 2014;8(2):119–22.
2. Adalja AA, Watson M, Bouri N, et al. Absorbing citywide patient surge during Hurricane Sandy: a case study in accommodating multiple hospital evacuations. Ann Emerg Med 2014;64(1):66–73.e1.
3. Tran CNT, Heller M, Berger A, et al. Hurricane Sandy: how did we do? Assessing a Manhattan Hospital's response. Front Public Health 2014;2:90.
4. Schultz CH, Koenig KL, Auf der Heide E. Benchmarking for hospital evacuation: a critical data collection tool. Prehosp Disaster Med 2005;20(5):331–42.
5. Teperman S. Hurricane Sandy and the greater New York health care system. J Trauma Acute Care Surg 2013;74(6):1401–10.
6. Lien C, Raimo J, Abramowitz J, et al. Community healthcare delivery post-Hurricane Sandy: lessons from a mobile health unit. J Community Health 2014; 39(3):599–605.
7. Gibbs L, Holloway C. Hurricane Sandy after action: report and recommendations to Mayor Michael R. Bloomberg. Hurricane Sandy after action: report and recommendations to Mayor Michael R Bloomberg, vol. 36. New York: The City of New York; 2013.
8. Caspers C, Smith SW, Seth R, et al. Observation services linked with an urgent care center in the absence of an emergency department: an innovative mechanism to initiate efficient health care delivery in the aftermath of a natural disaster. Disaster Med Public Health Prep 2016;10(3):405–10.
9. Claver M, Dobalian A, Fickel JJ, et al. Comprehensive care for vulnerable elderly veterans during disasters. Arch Gerontol Geriatr 2013;56(1):205–13.
10. Gray BH, Hebert K. Hospitals in Hurricane Katrina: challenges facing custodial institutions in a disaster. J Health Care Poor Underserved 2007;18(2):283–98.
11. Sternberg E, Lee GC, Huard D. Counting crises: US hospital evacuations, 1971-1999. Prehosp Disaster Med 2004;19(2):150–7.
12. Bagaria J, Heggie C, Abrahams J, et al. Evacuation and sheltering of hospitals in emergencies: a review of international experience. Prehosp Disaster Med 2009; 24(5):461–7.
13. Chavez CW, Binder B. A hospital as victim and responder: the Sepulveda VA Medical Center and the Northridge earthquake. J Emerg Med 1996;14(4):445–54.

14. Kellermann AL. Crisis in the emergency department. N Engl J Med 2006;355(13): 1300–3.
15. Warden G, Griffin R, Erickson S, et al. Hospital-based emergency care: at the breaking point 2006. Institute of Medicine. Hospital-Based Emergency Care: At the Breaking Point. Washington, DC: The National Academies Press; 2007.
16. Pearce A. Emergency medical services at the crossroads. British Association for Accident and Emergency Medicine; 2009.
17. Davies F. Emergency care for children: growing pains. British Association for Accident and Emergency Medicine; 2009.
18. Pines JM, Mullins PM, Cooper JK, et al. National trends in emergency department use, care patterns, and quality of care of older adults in the United States. J Am Geriatr Soc 2013;61(1):12–7.
19. Rudowitz R, Rowland D, Shartzer A. Health care in New Orleans before and after Hurricane Katrina. Health Aff 2006;25(5):w393–406.
20. Aldrich N, Benson WF. Disaster preparedness and the chronic disease needs of vulnerable older adults. Prev Chronic Dis 2008;5(1):A27.
21. Levin KL, Berliner M, Merdjanoff A. Disaster planning for vulnerable populations: leveraging Community Human Service Organizations direct service delivery personnel. J Public Health Manag Pract 2014;20:S79–82.
22. Arrieta MI, Foreman RD, Crook ED, et al. Insuring continuity of care for chronic disease patients after a disaster: key preparedness elements. Am J Med Sci 2008;336(2):128–33.
23. Sharma AJ, Weiss EC, Young SL, et al. Chronic disease and related conditions at emergency treatment facilities in the New Orleans area after Hurricane Katrina. Disaster Med Public Health Prep 2008;2(1):27–32.
24. Rosenblatt K. Nurses fleeing fast-moving camp fire scramble to save patients — and themselves 2018. Available at: https://www.nbcnews.com/news/us-news/nurses-fleeing-fast-moving-camp-fire-scramble-save-patients-themselves-n934961. Accessed December 03, 2018.
25. Nicas J. A melted Toyota tells the story of a brave nurse's actions during the California fires 2018. Availble at: https://twitter.com/i/moments/1062190467545092096?lang=en. Accessed December 03, 2018.
26. Lazar EJ, Cagliuso NV, Gebbie KM. Are we ready and how do we know? The urgent need for performance metrics in hospital emergency management. Disaster Med Public Health Prep 2009;3(1):57–60.
27. Abir M, Bell SA, Puppala N, et al. Setting foundations for developing disaster response metrics. Disaster Med Public Health Prep 2017;11(4):505–9.
28. Lurie N, Wasserman J, Nelson CD. Public health preparedness: evolution or revolution? Health Aff 2006;25(4):935–45.
29. Birnbaum ML. Accentuate the positive. Prehosp Disaster Med 2006;21(4):221–2.

Moving?

Make sure your subscription moves with you!

To notify us of your new address, find your **Clinics Account Number** (located on your mailing label above your name), and contact customer service at:

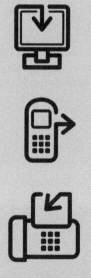

Email: journalscustomerservice-usa@elsevier.com

800-654-2452 (subscribers in the U.S. & Canada)
314-447-8871 (subscribers outside of the U.S. & Canada)

Fax number: 314-447-8029

Elsevier Health Sciences Division
Subscription Customer Service
3251 Riverport Lane
Maryland Heights, MO 63043

*To ensure uninterrupted delivery of your subscription, please notify us at least 4 weeks in advance of move.

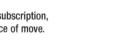

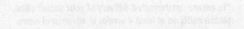

Printed and bound by CPI Group (UK) Ltd, Croydon, CR0 4YY

03/10/2024

01040483-0011